IN THE RE

Emily Parr

JANUS PUBLISHING COMPANY LTD
Cambridge, England

First published in Great Britain 2008
by Janus Publishing Company Ltd
The Studio
High Green
Great Shelford
Cambridge CB22 5EG

www.januspublishing.co.uk

Copyright © Emily Parr 2008

British Library Cataloguing-in-Publication Data
A catalogue record for this book is available from the British Library

ISBN 978-1-85756-634-5

All rights reserved. No part of this publication may be reproduced, stored in a retrieval system or transmitted in any form or by any means, electric, mechanical, photocopying, recording or otherwise, without the prior permission of the publisher.

The right of Emily Parr to be identified as the author of this work has been asserted by her in accordance with the Copyright, Designs and Patents Act 1988.

Cover Design: Kevin Mwangi

Printed and bound in the UK by PublishPoint
from KnowledgePoint Limited, Reading

Dedication

Calm seas do not make skilled sailors.
Flat roads do not make skilled mountain bikers,
but they do make some very happy marathon runners.

For Great Uncle Bill (Gubby) and Margaret Parr

Contents

Acknowledgements	ix
Prologue	xi
1. Might Be ...	1
2. Introducing Emily Parr	15
3. Hospital	17
4. The Next Bit	29
5. Mexico Coast-to-Coast Cycling Challenge; El Grandisimo	35
6. My Lesson Learned	67
7. Back to Life	71

Acknowledgements

Thanks to Macmillan Cancer Support and Tim, my Macmillan nurse; you mean a lot to me. Macmillan Cancer Support is a fantastic charity – it does a lot of vital work caring for people affected by cancer. Thanks to Cameron Fulljames for inspiring me to write my story.

Thanks to the National Health Service (NHS) and to all my doctors and nurses for looking after me. Thanks to my friends and family for supporting me in so many ways.

Thanks to Macmillan Cancer Support and Discover Adventure and Dr R for encouraging me to ride across Mexico, because we all believed in each other. Thanks to all of my private sponsors for the Mexico coast-to-coast challenge and to the Bryan Lancaster Trust for helping me to publish this book. Thanks to Amy, Les, Lindsey and Julie for checking my words. Thanks to whoever suggested that I publish this text as a book, I have forgotten who you are but it turns out that it was a great idea. Thanks to my publishers at Janus for all your hard work getting this book published and making me an author.

Thanks to Jon for making me smile when everything seemed pretty bleak. Thanks to everyone on Team Macmillan during El Grandisimo 2006. And a huge thanks to myself for surviving.

Prologue

This story is about a brain tumour, two bikes, some fear, some glory, a cat in England, several dogs in Mexico, a lot of courage and a very headstrong girl. This is a true story that happened to me; it was traumatic, devastating and eventually amazing, but life is full of epic things.

    I first wrote this book as a means of trying to understand my emotions regarding the experiences that I describe in this book and writing this very honest account proved to be incredibly therapeutic for me. A friend read it and suggested I make this into a book, to which I first thought "Nah" and then "Okay", and so here it is. I hope you benefit from reading the story as much as I did by living through it.

    In my opinion, the only thing that is guaranteed in life is change. Everything changes with the passage of time. For example, the experiences this book portrays seemed awfully tragic and negative when considered individually, but with the benefit of a constantly widening perspective and some passage of time, they seem like components of a bigger, more positive experience. Also lots of people say that time heals all wounds.

1

Might Be ...

I was twenty when I had my first cancer scare and after several months of tests, the results came back as negative and it was confirmed as a false alarm. I carried on doing a million things at university during that time and ran the London Marathon when I was twenty-one, which was evidence of how alive I was. I had just become twenty-two when I had my second cancer scare, when I was studying during the final year of my Modern Languages degree. This story is about the second time it happened to me. My life was exciting, intense and stressful, but mostly okay and fun. My issues were fairly typical for a student; food, boys, money, fun, work, clothes, rock climbing, snowboarding and the future.

I had always been aware that I had less hearing in my right ear than in my left one and it had never bothered me much up until then. I had never had a reason to question it before, but I was eager to have it checked out by a doctor, because any official notification of a hearing problem to my university could have boosted my marks. I was already doing well and getting excellent grades, but who'd say no to a free mark?

Not me, so in December 2004, I went to the local hospital for an audiology test.

The test consisted of me going into a little padded room, where they placed some headphones on me and I listened out for high-pitched squealing sounds and pressed a button whenever I heard one. After the test, my results showed on a graph on a computer screen. The audiologist conducting the test looked at me with suspicion as she informed me that there was a tiny hearing deficiency in my right ear when compared with my left one, but that there was nothing major wrong with my ears. She thought I was a fraud and I felt like grabbing her and shouting, "You're wrong!" I knew something was not right.

Next, I saw Dr P and he explained that he was sending me for an MRI (Magnetic Resonance Imaging Spectroscopy) scan to make sure I was okay. I didn't know what it was all about at the time and just felt grateful that the NHS was looking after me. Dr P said he was ninety-nine per cent sure it would be fine; little did I know how real and scary his one per cent of doubt would be. I left his office assuming that all would be fine.

I went back to my house in the student area of town, where I lived with a selection of people, who I thought were pretty miserable. It was hard work living with them and I do not even know where they are now. However, I lived with one cool girl called Olivia, who had been on the university rowing team with me a year beforehand. We got on well and were similarly energetic and overly conscientious. I liked it when she called me the "Bionic Woman".

One day in December 2004, I cycled off to the local hospital for my appointment for an MRI scan. I was on my beautiful, red vintage racer that I named "Big Red" – the bike was older than me and was falling apart with overuse. I was apprehensive about the scan because of my claustrophobia, knowing vaguely that MRI scans involved lying in a tight tunnel. When I shared this fear with Olivia on the morning of the scan, she offered to accompany me to the appointment, but I knew she was really busy at work and said no, effectively rejecting her support. I should have said yes, as by turning her offer down I was opting to be alone, blindly embarking on a terrifying journey.

However, I was not fully aware of the gravity of the situation at the time.

Arriving at the hospital, I walked confidently into the clinic waiting room, unperturbed by the other patients, who all seemed pretty old. I waited alone, flicking through a magazine

Might Be ...

or some university work, when my turn finally arrived. A male nurse led me out of the back door to a mobile MRI unit in a lorry. Inside it were two dark rooms partitioned by a big glass window and there were two radiographers, one Australian guy and one South African lady. We were all in one room, which was like the cockpit of a plane, with computer screens and flashing lights everywhere.

The Australian turned to me and said, 'Remove anything metal you're wearing and put it in the box on the side.' He was very friendly and pretty good-looking. Later, a nurse told me that MRI scanners are basically like huge electromagnets that create a magnetic force that is easily strong enough to throw a metal wheelchair across a room. So it would have ripped anything metal off me and sent it flying, which could have been very dangerous. So I took off all the metal things about my person and put them in the little red box. There were more items than I thought I had: my necklace, bracelets, toe-ring, hair elastic and hair clips.

The South African spoke next, saying, 'Could you be pregnant?'

'Er, no,' I said, thinking hard if I could be or not.

'Do you have metal in your eyes or head; shrapnel, for example?'

'Er,' I said, thinking hard again, even though I knew that I did not. Could some have snuck in there without me noticing it? 'No,' I answered cautiously.

'Have you had an MRI scan before?'

'No.'

The good-looking Australian took me into the other room, where there was a huge cylindrical machine on its side with a hole in the middle and a trolley extending out of the hole. 'Just take your shoes off and lie on this trolley,' he said.

I had a final thought, 'Oh, the rivets in my jeans are metal.'

'Ah, that's okay,' he replied.

I lay down, thinking how weird and sci-fi this all was. The Australian then handed me some protective earphones; I was confused, but put them on anyway. Next, he fitted my head on padding and placed a cage around it, restricting my movement.

I felt a huge pang of fear for the first time, as my head was trapped in a tiny space, causing major claustrophobia.

The Australian put a squeezer in my hand and reassured me, 'Just squeeze this if you want us to stop the scan at any time.'

Then he slid the trolley into the machine, until my head and shoulders were covered, at which point he left me alone in the room. I was lying flat on my back, with my head in a cage and my head and shoulders trapped in a tight tunnel. It was a claustrophobic nightmare, but I tried to stay calm. It felt wrong being trapped like that, but my rational side told me that I was safe and that this was probably all for my own good.

When I was younger, I was even more claustrophobic than I am now. I hated small spaces with a passion, especially when my big sisters trapped me in the cupboard under the stairs in our house or in a sleeping bag. I simply refused to go in lifts and remember once, at four years of age, screaming at my mum, when she tried to take me in one with my siblings. But now I am older, the feelings of claustrophobia have subsided as my sense of rationality has increased. I have learnt that I am probably safe in lifts, even though they still scare me a bit sometimes, and I know that the chances of it either crashing to the ground or me having a coughing fit and suffocating whilst inside it are very minimal. I got used to going in lifts when I lived in France in 2003. All French buildings seem to incorporate vast amounts of staircases and taking a lift multiple times a day is necessary to prevent oneself from becoming completely exhausted through the effort of climbing them all.

So I lay in the MRI machine, alone and trying not to worry too much. Then the noise of a pneumatic drill or a woodpecker began. The machine made lots of different noises, a cacophony of tapping and drilling sounds, and they seemed like a bizarre techno beat. This went on for several minutes; I was intrigued and had my eyes wide open. Then it was over, the Australian came back into the room, slid my trolley out of the machine and freed my head from the cage. I sat up immediately, glad to be out.

'How was that?' he asked, smiling.

Might Be ...

'Er, okay,' I answered, a bit spaced out. Then I put my blue Converse shoes on and followed him back to the first room we had started in. On the screens were lots of cross-sectioned images of my skull and brain. Wow! This was the first time I had ever seen my brain. I had spent my whole life being so close to it, relying on it, using it to think and exist, and yet I had never seen it until then. Maybe we are not supposed to see those things, as seeing a supernatural being may not be an everyday event, nature certainly does not grow MRI scanners. Seeing my brain for the first time excited me.

'What's this? And this?' I asked, pointing at the pictures.

'Does it look okay?' I was like a child at Christmas time.

'We can't discuss the images with you,' said the South African drily.

'Oh, okay,' I said, feeling rather disappointed. They looked okay to me, how did I not see the oh-so-obvious grey blurry "not okay" patch.

The Australian handed me my metal stuff and it took a couple of minutes for me to put it all back on. 'We'll process your results and send you a letter in three weeks' time,' said one of the nurses.

'Okay, is that all?' I said, wondering if I could have a printout of my brain images, but not daring to ask for one.

Instead, I said, 'Thanks,' and left the building to cycle the short distance back to university, without wearing my cycling helmet.

I did not think the scan was that big a deal and on 4 January 2005, I went snowboarding in the French Alps for a week with the university snow-sports club. It was my first snowboarding trip and was a lot of fun, although I spent the majority of the time falling on my arse and the rest of the time getting drunk with a bunch of students I found to be quite socially awkward.

On a snowboard, I could turn and go fast, but I could not control myself or stop without pain, so that week I bumped and bruised my body and head more times than I care to remember in such a short space of time. That is to say, that this week was particularly bad for me, when compared with the huge amounts of pain I'd experienced as a teenager, frequently by falling off ramps and stuff whilst skating. It was on this trip that I met Justine at the bar one evening. She always wore a headscarf and when I asked her about her hair, she said it was a wig, as she'd had cancer before and had lost some hair as a result of the chemotherapy treatment. As we chatted, I found her to be inspirational; it reminded me of Lance Armstrong's story, *It's Not About the Bike*, in which he recalls how he overcame cancer and went on to win the Tour de France. In my opinion, he is a champion cyclist, and I thought Justine was likewise both amazing and honest, but I never imagined how closely it might relate to me in later months.

Years later, I found out that Lance Armstrong's success post-cancer had been a drug-fuelled lie. I felt betrayed to know how hollow he really was and how I had eagerly believed him to be an incredible inspiration.

Back at home in the UK, the expected letter was waiting for me. It said I was to go to the ENT (Ear, Nose and Throat) department of my local hospital on 24 January 2005 for my MRI scan results. I took a deep breath – D-Day (Diagnosis-day).

I rode there on my bike, in a state of anxiety – after all, isn't everyone anxious about results, until they hear that it's all okay? In the doctor's office were a doctor and another guy called Tim from Macmillan Cancer Support (a charity previously called Macmillan Cancer Relief). I was a bit freaked out at seeing two men waiting for me, but decided it must be a matter of routine.

The doctor told me straight, 'The results of your scan show a tumour in your ear.' I was not shocked, they were simply confirming the existence of my hearing difficulty and quite naively, I felt relieved, as they legitimised my feelings of anxiety. The doctor introduced me to the other guy, 'This is Tim and he's a cancer support nurse.'

What! I thought; this situation was escalating way too fast.

'Cancer? But I don't have cancer; you said a moment ago that it's just a tumour in my ear, not cancer.'

Might Be ...

I followed Tim into a different room, where we sat down together. Tim had a gentle voice and he said, 'You don't have cancer; I am a cancer specialist, but I deal with anyone who has an abnormal growth in their head region.' We talked about university and family and ear tumours for a while, while I desperately avoided crying and tried to keep a brave face, but it felt like my guts were being ripped out and burnt in front me.

Tim eventually said, 'We'll be in touch soon about further treatment, I mean within days. I think you'll find the NHS moves quite fast at this level of urgency.'

I cycled off and don't remember what I did that night, probably some university work to try and distract me. However, what I do know is that I was thanking my lucky stars that the tumour was in my ear and not in my brain. I felt that had it been in my brain, I would have been screwed; it might as well have been a death sentence as far as I was concerned.

The next day, I woke up feeling quite positive about the diagnosis. The news was bad, but it could have been so much worse. Little did I know that the events that were about to unfold would change my life immensely and horrifically. I went to the university library in the morning to study for a few hours – I worked obsessively hard at university and put in all the hours I could – and I then went to my grandparents' house for lunch. They conveniently lived a ten-minute bike ride from my university campus and I visited them several times a week to get fed and to help them do their shopping. More importantly, I got the love and support that only grandparents can offer and they loved having me around too. I really enjoyed seeing them so often; we have always been really close.

I was having my customary post-lunch nap during a visit to my grandparents' house, when I received a voice message on my mobile. It was my GP, Dr R at the university health centre.

Dr R said, 'Emily, please call the health centre as soon as you get this message.' So I went downstairs and used my grandparents' landline to call him as, predictably, I had no credit left on my mobile. Dr R said, 'Hi, Emily, can you come to the practice please?' He spoke in an urgent tone.

'When?' I asked.

'Now would be good,' he answered emphatically.

So I forgot any ideas of chilling out and grabbed my bike, riding fast to the health centre

On entering, I told the receptionist who I was and after a very short wait in a rather full waiting room, Dr R appeared, all smiles as usual; he was a really nice guy who I liked. 'Hi, Emily, come through to my office,' he said. However, that day, his smile was one of grim determination.

After putting down the phone and before sitting down in his office, I had assumed the news to be positive and that progress had been made already in sorting out the minor problem of my ear tumour. But as I entered Dr R's office, I saw that Tim was there again and remember thinking that he seemed to turn up everywhere. We all sat down and their chairs were in front of me. Tim's expression was completely serious and I felt a bit nervous, but generally optimistic. After the door was closed, we got straight down to the business of destroying reality as I knew it.

Tim spoke first. 'After I met you yesterday, I thought it best to get your scan results rechecked, so that's what I did. I'm afraid that the tumour isn't in your ear.' The ear tumour that I had felt vaguely grateful to for not being in my brain had never existed.

Dr R continued for him and his words have defined everything in my experience since he spoke. He said, 'It's in your brain. Emily, I'm so sorry.'

Tim watched and my reaction was calm on the outside, but something deep inside me screamed "No!" I could not believe it. I was used to things in life being more or less okay, but this was not cool and neither was it anything I had ever envisaged hearing. It was not part of my script, so I just stared at the wall over the doctor's right shoulder. I waited for someone to unsay it, or say that it wasn't true, that it was all just a sick joke, but no one spoke and whilst I was staring into space, I wasn't really looking at anything in particular. Inside, I felt my heart was being dragged violently down into my stomach by twenty lorries. Fireworks went off behind my eyes and a baseball bat slammed repeatedly against my head as my breath burned and parts of me began to melt. I was completely stunned. Dr R may as well have told me I was dying, as I feel that it might have caused me to have a similar reaction.

Tim watched me in silence and when he got no obvious reaction, he prompted, 'Emily, are you okay? You're being a little too cool for my liking.'

I responded in a clumsy, floundering stammer, 'Yeh, erm, I'm fine, erm … actually, it's as if you've got a baseball bat and hit me really hard on the head, I'm shocked.' I threw my gaze around the doctor's office.

'I'm sorry,' Dr R offered again in a gentle voice, but I didn't feel upset at first. It hadn't fully sunk in. All they knew was that I had a tumour in my brain, they didn't know what kind it was, whether it was benign or malignant, big or small, cancer or not, and they certainly couldn't tell me if it would kill me or not, which was what I really wanted to know. Dr R broke into my thoughts and said, 'You'll be sent for a biopsy next and we'll be in touch soon to let you know when the hospital appointment is booked for.'

Internally, I was confused. Hospital, biopsy, what? Hospital, biopsy, what? I had never been to hospital before and had no idea what a biopsy entailed, although I guessed it was some sort of medical procedure. My memories of the next few minutes are hazy. Tim asked me what I would do that evening and I said I would probably see my friends or something. We shook hands and I flew down the corridor and out of the health centre.

Unlocking my bike, I decided that I couldn't go back to the loneliness of the student halls, so I left the university campus and rode the ten-minute journey across a park to my grandparents' house. Some time during that ride, I started sobbing with fear; it was overwhelming and I'm surprised that I managed to ride at all, without crashing or falling off my bike, as my eyes were full of tears.

I propped my bike up as normal behind the dilapidated shed in my grandparents' garden. The back door was unlocked and I walked straight into the kitchen. My grandma was there and I didn't say anything at first; all I could manage was to cry and hug her tightly for ages.

Finally, I said quietly, 'I've got a brain tumour.'

Earlier that day, I had explained to my grandparents about the ear tumour situation, which had scared me at the time, but not nearly as much as this new information did. The earlier explanation had been tearless and yet I felt everything had ramped up a notch or two since then. My grandma knew just how to comfort me and eventually I stopped crying and she asked, 'Do you want to phone your mother?'

I remember wanting to be alone when I phoned my mum and I have no recollection of having anything to eat that evening, but at some point, I cycled back to my room in my flat in university halls, housing students from all over the world. I sat crying and alone in my room, with my legs dangling off the bed like a kid, before plucking up the courage and stamina to contact a couple of people on my mobile. I had a conversation with my mum that I imagine no parent ever wants to have with their child. Most of the time, it's the parent that goes first; that's just how the world turns. It wasn't supposed to happen like this.

'Mum, I've got a brain tumour,' I managed to squeeze out between my tears.

She was very calm and I'm grateful to her for that. We talked for a while and I asked her to call my sisters and brother with the bad news, as I couldn't face doing it myself. I naturally thought of Justine, the girl who I had met on the university snow-sports trip a couple of months earlier. I didn't know her that well, but sent her a text message to tell her my news. I felt sure that she would understand and she did, she rang me back immediately and was so sweet and compassionate that words fail me.

She asked what I had been told and said, 'Where are you? I'm coming round.'

Might Be ...

Conveniently, she lived on the university campus five minutes from me and I felt slightly relieved that I was not going to be facing this alone. I was wearing a red hoody and when she knocked at the door of my flat, I let her in and cried relentlessly. She gave me a massive hug and we talked about my day and of what I did and did not know. We discussed what would happen next and although I did not really know, it scared me more than one can imagine. Justine was awesome, extremely pragmatic and totally reassured me that everything was going to be okay; she had lost close members of her family to cancer and had survived the illness herself twice.

She was a medical student and knew what it was that we needed to do. 'We need information,' she said, 'I'll sort that for you.' She instinctively knew where to look and what to do and ultimately took control of the situation when I was a gibbering wreck. In hindsight, I feel it's obvious why I'd had that conversation with her at the bar in France about her cancer.

Although I never suspected it would be hugely beneficial to me at the time, I think it happened so that she could help me – call it fate, if you like. Over the next few weeks and months, Justine proved to be a great friend and was very supportive. Because of her own experiences, she knew just the right things to do and say to reassure and help me. She left that night giving me another huge hug and looking sympathetically at my distressed face, promising to call the next day. Alone again, I cried even more that night and found it hard to sleep, something I was going to have to come to terms with over the next few months.

The next few days proved harder than I could ever have imagined. I tried to concentrate on university work, but it was a bad way to try and distract myself, as the work was so intense.

I was supposed to be completing the degree course with my classmates in a matter of weeks and whilst the workload was harsh, I had felt just about able to handle it all. However, I had seen my university tutor Dr B a few weeks previously and had explained that various factors in my personal life had combined to add extra stress and I'd admitted that I was finding it difficult to concentrate on my work. These problems were dwarfed by the discovery of the brain tumour, after which I emailed my university adviser Madame T and asked for Special Consideration, due to my epic anxiety. Needless to say, I got it, although I was unable to talk to her in person about my medical issues, for fear of breaking down and crying, and that was the last thing I wanted.

Justine called and gave me various sheets of information on brain tumours that she'd found on the Internet. We met up quite a lot and she talked sensibly to me, nearly convincing me that I might be okay. 'Read this,' she said.

The paper stated that, "Over fifty per cent of brain tumours are not cancerous; many of these are benign and never present a medical problem."

Perhaps I was one of those cases. Perhaps I could conceivably survive. It was really comforting to think this way and, in fact, this new information was more encouraging and inspirational than anything the professional medics had told me. What they had told me was very general in terms of, 'You have a brain tumour.' This could have meant anything to a non-medic like me so my instinctive reaction was to jump to the conclusion that I was dying. It is human nature for an ignorant person to assume the worst scenario in a bad situation and this felt like one such situation; indeed, it was the worst situation that I had ever been in.

Ever since leaving the health centre, all I could think about were Dr R's words, 'We'll call you', flying around in my head and Tim's advice to keep my phone with me at all times. I was constantly waiting for a call and my phone was never far away from me; I slept with it at my side, I left it on in my pocket in the library and I even took it into the kitchen and the bathroom with me. You name it, it went there. I was determined not to miss such an important call, as if it was some sort of lifeline. The call finally came after ten days of waiting and in those days, I tried to get on with my university work with little success, as I was wracked with anxiety, trying desperately to get used to this menacing new idea. During this time, I told some close friends about what was happening to me. I was comforted by some of their responses and both confused and disappointed by others. Olivia said, 'Oh my god,' Francesca and Tom said, 'We'll get it sorted,' and Elsa comforted, 'It'll be okay, Em.' Others made me angry by saying, 'I'm sure you'll be fine,' as if I'd just told them I had a common cold or some other minor ailment. Sometimes I talked to my mum, sometimes to my siblings. I cannot remember what we said, but concerns were voiced, tears were shed and pain was expressed.

Everyone in the family hurt; me, my parents, my two big sisters, my twin brother and my grandparents. It was nice that the family drew together in a crisis. We were collectively scared and yet, I felt that I was the only one really suffering, with the reality of this alien in my head, and that it was only I who could realistically consider the scary prospects that lay ahead. Despite all this communication between us, it was a very difficult and lonely time; a tiny preview of what lay in store for me.

I was referred to see Mr L the neurosurgeon at the local hospital in the oncology department, which was full of hairless cancer patients. I was terrified and wrote in my diary: He asked me loads of questions about my symptoms. I told him I often get dizzy when doing sports and that my sense of balance isn't very good. I told him I really liked rowing, because it is a tough sport that you sit down to do and that rowers can't fall over, because they are already sitting down on their bums. I told him all about my dodgy eyesight, my hearing and my ambidextrous skills; writing right-handed, but using cutlery and playing pool left-handed. He checked my reflexes with a hammer, touched the skin on my face with pins to ascertain my sensitivity and even scratched my feet. He made me touch my nose and then his index finger, which he moved back and forth constantly to check my coordination and then he checked my balance, I had to stand with my feet together, which was hard. He said I was remarkably well, but needed more scans. I remember thinking to myself that whatever the outcome, I just needed courage and conviction and it was with this in mind that I hoped it would all get sorted.

Tim called a few days later. I was in bed at the time and answered the phone almost instantly.

'That was quick,' he mused.

'The phone was right next to me,' I replied, not amused.

Tim was a lovely nurse who was sent to look after me from Macmillan Cancer Support. He told me a bed was free in a few days time at one of the UK's specialist neuroscience hospitals, which was relatively close to my university town. The appointment was for another MRI scan and a biopsy, but it was not for a few days yet, so that afternoon I went rock climbing and in the evening I partied. Over the next few days, I watched films and dreamed of going somewhere sunny and of living life to the full.

2

Introducing Emily Parr

Throughout my life I have generally been healthy and successful. Although I have experienced illness and tragedy, I had a stable, happy family life when I was younger, with two parents, two older sisters and a twin brother. Everything stemmed from my positive experience of family life. Our hometown was in northern England, where I lived until I left for university at eighteen years of age. My whole life was joyful and easy and I had lots of friends and lots of fun. I'd always got excellent grades at school and was on all the school sports teams. I sang in the school choir, played in the school orchestra and wind band and acted in the school's drama club.

I played both the French horn and the piano at Grade 5 standard (the Associated Board of the Royal Schools of Music certificates), I played the guitar and trumpet and I had also enjoyed being part of two samba bands. At eighteen years old, I gained my Gold Duke of Edinburgh's award, a Community Sports Leadership award, a blue belt in karate and I was very proud to hold a full, clean driving licence. I enjoyed raising funds for charity and had also gone abroad to take part in some international voluntary work-camp projects, helping in several challenged communities.

In my teenage years, I was very involved in organising and participating in local and national events for a big youth organisation.

I had done loads of jobs to earn some extra cash, from waitressing and childcare, to technical operator in the local radio station. At university, I was part of the rowing team and the sports representative of my school, as well as secretary of the French society. As part of my Modern Languages degree, I lived and studied in France for a year, returning to the UK in April 2004 to run the London Marathon, raising thousands of pounds for charity. I came back from France and started studying for my final year at university, when I had my initial audiology test and life got scary. I'm extremely proud that I got a 2:1 classification for my degree, despite all this stressful medical stuff happening to me at the time.

3

Hospital

Friday 4 March 2005. Day One:

It was snowing heavily and the thin tyres on "Big Red", my bike, wouldn't grip the road, so I cursed Mother Nature and walked to my grandparents' house instead. I hoped the snow would stop or the roads would be screwed up, so that my mum and I wouldn't be able to drive to the hospital, thereby messing up our plans. But it stopped snowing and Mum was able to take me, because I didn't have a car. We arrived at hospital at 2.00 p.m. with a family friend and waited for two hours, watching television in the visitors' day room. Eventually, a nurse came, took a blood sample from me and said I could leave and come back on the Sunday night, ready for my scan on the Monday.

She explained that this was because lots of doctors were off at the weekend and that I was not booked into theatre until Wednesday. The operating theatre? I wondered. Maybe she thinks I'm here for an operation. At this point, I still didn't understand what a biopsy entailed, so I booked into my bed and was glad to be let out for the weekend, because I didn't relish the thought of staying in hospital very much.

Saturday 5 March 2005. Day Two:

I went back to a friend's house and was very tense and irritable.

I wrote in my diary: I am alone. We all are. I feel like it's an insight into how superficial a lot of human interaction is. It's full of shit. I continued: I've curled up, clenched my fists, screwed up my face, cried and cried, clenched my teeth, wished it wasn't me, put my head in the crack between the pillow and the wall, wishing it would disappear, sat in the darkness of the cinema and willed the film never to end. I just want to throw something hard and run really fast, faster than I ever have before. How can you tell me this? I'm twenty-two. I'm really healthy.

Sunday 6 March 2005. Day Three:

I arrived at hospital and checked into my ward in the evening.

A nurse showed me to my bed and as I entered, the other patients in my ward stared at me. They were scary, like a collection of broken toys, horrific but harmless, with varying degrees of hair loss. I was at a loss as to what to do with myself; I felt reluctant to put on my pyjamas and act like a real hospital patient or a really ill person, so I sat on the bed fully clothed. A nurse told me to remove all my jewellery and she put an ID bracelet displaying my hospital number on each of my wrists. Later, I found out that ID bracelets are put on both of the patient's wrists, so that if they die on the operating table, they are easily identifiable. Dr H the house doctor came to see me a short while later. I explained how I was about to finish my university degree and that this diagnosis couldn't have come at a worse time for me. She wisely pointed out that no time was a good time to get a diagnosis of this sort and I liked her way of thinking, because it was true. That night, my blood pressure was 110/70 and a blood test showed my blood was healthy, with good levels of minerals. When the nurses looked at me, their eyes seemed to say "Why are you here?" because I looked perfectly healthy; they were used to working with sick people. I don't know, was my silent reply.

The other five ladies on my ward all appeared to be a minimum of thirty years older than me. One lady, who I named the Bad Doll, stared at me constantly and openly throughout my stay in hospital. She was probably thinking, she's so young.

Another lady screamed "Ow, ow" all that night, whilst another cried and vomited noisily. Most of them had their heads shaved or half shaved. Shit, I thought, hair loss and the thought of dying terrified me. I came to refer to the hospital as the "half-hair hotel", as I thought I would lose half my hair and be forced to scream in pain like them. It was my first night in hospital and I felt very alone. After my mum had left, the nurse drew the curtain around my bed, but all night I could hear the lady's pained screams and profuse vomiting. I was scared and put my huge headphones on to try and drown out the noise.

Monday 7 March 2005. Day Four:
The impressively efficient nurses checked up on me many times a day:

	6.10 a.m.	10.55 a.m.	3.10 p.m.	7.40 p.m.	9.55 p.m.
Blood Pressure	106/65	113/71	121/82	111/71	120/74
Heartbeats Per Minute	72	82	90	80	80
Temperature °C	36.6	37.1	37.3	37.4	37.2
Blood Oxygenation Levels %	100	99	100	100	100

I wrote everything down about what they were doing, thinking it was important to record all the things that they were doing to me. I was constantly reviewing what I knew about my situation and wondering in terms of how I could improve it. In my diary, I wrote: It's in my brain stem and cerebellum at the back of my neck. Apparently, it'll be hard to remove and it's impossible to treat it with chemotherapy. But radiotherapy might be possible.

But must keep spirits up, can't stress that enough. All signs are good so far, except for the obvious, that is. Blood tests good, blood pressure good, blood one hundred per cent oxygenated – what more could I want?

Tom, my twin, called me on the phone; it was good to talk. He had not been able to visit the hospital that week, but promised to come as soon as he could the following weekend. It was a massive shame that he could not visit me in the half-hair hotel; he was a great comfort to me and a good source of distraction. Tom is a wonderful person.

I had a stealth MRI scan to create a 3D image of the contents of my head. Before the scan, a doctor came and marked my skull with "Polos". These are small adhesive discs roughly 1 cm in diameter. They are stuck to the patient's skull during the scan to enable doctors to ascertain exactly where to cut into the person's head. However, this necessitated shaving tiny bits of my hair off, where they were to be positioned. I was terrified, but allowed the doctor to get on with whatever was necessary; what other alternative did I have?

A nurse came to the foot of my bed with a wheelchair to escort me to my scan two floors away. She was a bit chubby and I was insulted and felt indignant. I thought, I'm probably healthier than you and you have the nerve to offer me a wheelchair; but, instead, I said, 'I'll walk.'

She replied, 'Okay, if you think you can manage it.'

I gave her a demeaning glance and replied with a silent but scathing, 'Of course I can, you fucking idiot, I'm perfectly healthy.'

I walked to the scan in my blue flip flops, tartan pyjama trousers and red hoody. The MRI scan was almost identical to the one I'd had before at the hospital near my university, with the very same cacophony of drilling and tapping in a bizarre techno beat. My mum was allowed to stay with me during this scan and held my hand as I lay on the trolley, with my head once more trapped in a cage. This was a super MRI scan, the height of technology, creating a 3D image of my skull, whereas normal MRI scans only create a 2D image. For this scan to work, the nurse injected me with invisible dye, which would show up on my scan images. It's just as well that I didn't mind injections, because I was having rather a lot of them.

Hospital

After the scan, it was necessary to keep the "Polos" exactly where they were, until after the biopsy operation, leaving me feeling like an android, due to their apparent visibility. I cried a lot that day, while Mum hugged me and held my hand. It had become apparent to me that having a biopsy meant that I had to have some form of brain surgery. My biopsy was investigative surgery, to allow them to obtain cells from the brain tumour for pathologists and oncologists to analyse, rather than being removal of the tumour itself. My chief consultant and neurosurgeon had been changed from Mr L to Mr W, so that the biopsy could be done on Wednesday 9 March 2005. I was petrified and felt it totally unjustified that this was happening at all.

At 10.50 p.m., I took my first little white tablet of the catabolic steroid dexamethasone and another pill for stomach protection called lansoprazole. Looks can be deceiving and whilst these steroid tablets were small and white, looking innocent and harmless, I grew to hate them very strongly, very quickly.

Tuesday 8 March 2005. Day Five:

	6.50 a.m.
Blood Pressure	117/61
Heart Rate in beats per minute	100
Temperature °C	36
Blood Oxygenation level %	100

I'd had a dream the previous night that I was given four steroid tablets to take and I just couldn't swallow them for the life of me. A nurse was teaching me how to swallow in the dream, which I later recalled when they brought me two steroid pills and a stomach protection pill at 7.30 a.m.

After various medical checks in the morning, I was allowed to leave the hospital for the afternoon. I put on normal, civilian clothes and my mum and I walked around a pretty country garden by a river; I hardly even saw it. We ate soup in the café there and I felt painfully conscious of the "Polos" stuck on my head, feeling and looking every bit a sick person.

I returned to the hospital with my mum that evening, when I changed back into my pyjamas and got back on my bed. We sat reading until 10.00 p.m., when a young doctor came to see me. He explained about the biopsy that I would have the next morning and exactly what the surgery entailed. He stressed how dangerous it was and that there was a 10–15 per cent chance that the surgery would go wrong, causing a stroke, a brain haemorrhage, an infection in my brain or even my death.

However, he reassured me that the actual chances of me dying would be less than one per cent. Oh cheers, mate! He then apologised and presented me with a legal form to sign, declaring that I had understood all of the stuff he'd said, sort of like a contract, and then he handed me a pen.

Gripped by fear, I glanced at my mum, who nodded and said quietly, 'I think you'll have to.' So I duly signed it, although it all felt so wrong, like I was signing my own death warrant. She signed as a witness of the process and then the doctor left. With the curtain drawn around the bed, we were both petrified and crying as we held each other in mutual mixed feelings of emotion. Mum just hugged me tightly, 'I love you, Emily,' she said, while I just thought, Oh shit, I am going to die. She left a short while later and the young doctor came back with a razor in his hand; he had come to shave my hair off ready for surgery and he was very apologetic about this whole thing as well.

Looking down, I bent my neck forwards and he dry-shaved three square inches of my four inch long hair off the back of my head. It sounded like ripping Velcro. I was petrified and had never valued my hair as much as I did in that moment, when I seriously thought I might lose it all. I vowed that if I had any left when I got out of hospital, I would be nicer to it and not always shove it up in a scruffy ponytail like I normally did.

Hospital

Tim said I was lucky to lose only that much hair, because three decades earlier, all brain surgery patients had had their heads completely shaven.

I had been told I was nil-by-mouth and that I was not to eat or drink anything from midnight until after the operation the next morning. With this in mind, I felt that it was important to consume as much as I could in the little time available to me. I watched some extreme motocross on television and stuffed my face with chocolate and grapes, drinking Ribena as I did so.

On the stroke of midnight, I downed my drink and surrendered my remaining food to the nurse. I then listened to some music by Modest Mouse, as my friend Davina had recommended that I listen to track three – *And we'll all float on okay*. Ironic really. I was worried about getting thirsty and having a fatal coughing fit before the operation, my imagination running away with the fear and anxiety of it all, although this fear was very real.

It is harrowing to remember thinking seriously about dying and in my diary that night, I wrote a short will for my family, in case of the worst. I was very pragmatic about it all. I called two people on the phone that night, my twin brother Tom and my friend Kate. I was in floods of tears in my bed, whilst at the same time trying to be quiet, so as not to disturb the rest of the ward. I'm sure I had nothing to say really, except perhaps, 'I think I might die tomorrow.' I could not talk to Kate for long, because she was in America and my international phonecard ran out. In my diary I wrote: I'll be okay; I'm a warrior, and I'll be okay.

Wednesday 9 March 2005. Day Six:

I was woken by a nurse at 6.00 a.m. She handed me a surgery gown and anti-blood-clotting socks. The socks were long and tight and the gown was massive and opened at the back. They were all white, like an angel's outfit or huge death garments.

The ID bracelets were still on my wrists and the "Polos" were still stuck on my head. At 8.00 a.m., I was wheeled into the operating theatre in my bed; the nurses didn't give me the option of walking, so I didn't mention it. I felt a bit like a fraud, because I could have walked there. Three anaesthetists put me to sleep and the anaesthetic was delivered by injecting it into the back of my hand through a tube. Someone had told me to count from ten down to one, by which time I would be asleep.

I was anxious to get it over with and lay in that bright room thinking, oh God, will I wake up? And if I do, will I be the same? I counted from ten down to one, but I was still awake. An anaesthetist said, 'Not yet, not yet,' so I counted up from one to ten, but again I was still awake, so I began counting from ten down to one again, when the anaesthetist eventually said, 'You might taste plastic in the back of your throat.' I did, and passed out at the count of six.

I woke up in the bright recovery room and immediately said, 'But you didn't even…' Touching the back of my head I felt a huge dressing there. I was shocked and had no recollection of the past two hours even having existed. But, apparently, they had and someone had been sticking sharp things into my head.

It did not seem like the normal definition of sleep, after which you know that time has passed, even though you were unconscious. It was the ultimate strange feeling for me to wake up without any awareness of having been asleep. People in white masks were staring at me and I had a huge, induced head injury that I had no intention of having and no recollection of receiving.

One of the anaesthetists told me to squeeze her hand, press down with my feet and blink my eyes. I chattered incessantly as the nurse wheeled me back to the ward, and she laughed, 'Are you high, Emily? Because they gave you morphine in there.'

I heard that and instantly decided I needed more. 'I need more morphine. I need more morphine,' I said. It's funny, because I don't like hard drugs under normal circumstances.

Back on the ward, I was given a painkiller that was less powerful than morphine and I fell asleep. I cannot remember much of that day, but when I woke up, my mum was by my bed

Hospital

and I glanced at the sheet beneath my head. There was blood spattered on it and I remember thinking that it must have been mine, but I didn't react at all. My neck muscles hurt so much.

Some of them had been cut in surgery like guy ropes on a tent and it meant that moving my head at all required me to put my hands underneath it and lift it. I kept finding sensor pads, plasters and catheters stuck all over my body throughout the day on my legs, arms, back and stomach. I thought this was good, because it meant they had been checking up on me. My face was completely yellow from the antiseptic they'd used, like one of the Simpsons, and my throat was rough and dry. It was very sore and I was sure that they must have shoved a tube in there at some point during the operation.

Mr W my surgeon came to see me with a gaggle of doctors and nurses. I sat up with some difficulty and shook his hand. 'Did you get a picture of my brain?' I asked immediately.

'No,' he replied.

I was slightly disappointed, thinking "Well what was the point in any of that operation?" and fell asleep again immediately, waking up a while later to find my dad was there.

The nurses' check ups became more frequent and diligent: they woke me, took my blood pressure, squeezed my hands and feet, asked me where I was, took my heart rate, temperature, blood oxygenation level and shone a bright torch in my eyes to check my pupil dilation. I hated them shining a torch in my eyes, when all I wanted to do was sleep, and my blood oxygenation level apparently fell to ninety-six per cent. When I woke up, my mum was there and then my sister arrived. I lifted my head with my hands and made a completely sick joke about having had a stroke in surgery, smiling at my sister with only half of my face.

'Oh, Emy, don't,' she said sternly, obviously horrified by my humour.

I stopped, secretly pleased not to have suffered a stroke and feeling thankful to have woken from the surgery at all. I felt grateful to the NHS doctors and nurses for looking after me.

When the young "head-shaving" doctor came back to see me later that day, I gave him a huge smile, kicking my legs, stretching my fingers open and then clenching my fists shut as a greeting, so that he could instantly see that I was fine and not paralysed.

That day, I was put on a high dosage of steroids to reduce brain swelling. I was to take four tablets several times daily – four steroid tablets, just like in my dream of the previous night. I woke in the evening. The drugs had made me ravenous, so I ate mashed potatoes, pasta and cake and then went back to sleep again.

The nurses checked me throughout the night and I was woken frequently, with the now customary squeeze of my hands and a torch being shone directly into my eyes.

Thursday 10 March 2005. Day Seven:

A cleaner came to put some clean sheets on my bed early in the morning. I had been sleeping and was annoyed; I waited in a nearby chair, still very high and disorientated from the drugs, and before she had finished doing my bed, I'd decided that it would be a good idea to go and check my email on the free Internet service in the hospital reception area a few floors below. I found the nurses at their desk in my ward and told them where I would be going, pledging to come back soon. For some reason, they agreed very quickly to my departure and I looked at them for a moment with glazed eyes and then gave them the most sickly-sweet smile that has ever passed across my face. I walked out of the ward slowly, not understanding why they had let me go. Maybe they thought I was fine. Once out of the ward, there was no one around in the corridor and I collapsed against a wall, dragged myself back up to my feet, found a lift and crumpled against the wall in there, too.

Somehow, I found a computer and managed to access my email account. I sent a very dark email about death to lots of my friends and then found my way back up to my ward and my freshly made bed. Nurses came round the ward with drugs; I took four steroid tablets, but refused any painkillers.

Hospital

'You have an extremely high tolerance to pain,' remarked the nurse.

Another nurse had already commented on my astonishingly high blood oxygenation levels. They were impressed with me; I thought nothing of it and slept all day, in between various visits from family, in addition to doctors and nurses' checking up on me at odd intervals.

That evening, I was discharged from hospital. The pharmacist came to see me and explained all about the medication I should take. I was given a big bag of drugs, including steroids and strong painkillers. The reduction of the steroid dose was explained to me and I was urged to take the painkillers at the first sign of any pain.

We drove away from the hospital slowly in dense traffic and the car jumped along, making my neck really hurt, which made me angry. It seemed as if the car gravitated into every single pothole on the way home.

4

The Next Bit

A lot of "The Next Bit" happened as if I was in some sort of a whirlwind and I have forgotten much of it, which is good, because it was horrible. I spent the first few days resting in the back bedroom at my sister's house, communicating with my mum and sister by text message to order drinks and food, etc.

I saw Tom that weekend and he hugged me tightly and said, 'We'll still go to New York,' as I had planned to run the New York Marathon to fund-raise for a charity. Underneath, I think he was as scared as me that we would never be able to do anything like that together again.

I then went to my grandparents' house with my mum for a few days. All this time, I was taking steroids and was pretty out of it. I was never in pain, but I liked the super-strength painkillers the hospital had given me. When I took them, they made me feel happy and light-headed and when I shut my eyes, they gave me the illusion that I was sleeping, which was good, as I was already feeling depressed and having lots of trouble sleeping. My driving licence had been automatically revoked after surgery and I lost it for six months. Many aspects of my identity had been challenged: my jewellery removed, my hair shaved off, my health questioned and my driving licence revoked. These things were stolen from me and it hurt a lot.

I saw Tim and Dr R a short while later. The steroids had caused me to get spots all over my face, which was hideous, so Dr R prescribed me with an antibiotic to sort the problem out, but it only made it much worse, which added to my feelings of gloom.

All this time, we were waiting for results to tell us about the prognosis of the tumour and whether I would live or die.

Unfortunately, all the hospital's pathologists were on their Easter holidays and the analysis of my results was delayed. It was critical information and I was being forced to wait to find out if I might die, all because people were on holiday getting a tan – it seemed desperately unfair.

On the day my mum drove us home to northern England, the hospital registrar rang my mobile phone. He said, 'I just thought I'd tell you, I can't say officially, but your results look okay. The tumour's benign and not cancerous. I just thought you'd want to know.'

I felt incredibly relieved, but the only celebration I could manage was to put my feet in the compartment under the glove box of the car. A few weeks later, those results were officially confirmed – they said the tumour was not cancer yet, but that it had the capacity to become cancerous later on. They said it was very rare for someone so young and healthy like me to have a condition like this, but that revelation did not make me feel very special at all.

Being at home all the time was depressing and I was very bored, with nothing to do. I had chronic insomnia and did not sleep for a month. My heart beat very quickly and loudly and I was unable to slow it down with calm breathing techniques and I could hear it all the time. Ten minutes would pass as slowly as ten years. Every day at 5.00 p.m. for a month, I had a panic attack lasting for about an hour on each occasion. During the attacks, I got really cold and shivered violently, but it was an internal coldness and blankets did nothing to warm me up. I believed I was going to die each time, I felt truly awful and even thought a few times that I would prefer to be dead than to endure these attacks any more. I tried to distract myself with music and films and walking with friends, but it was all merely efforts at temporary distraction and I still felt completely terrible underneath it all. When I was taking the steroids I had no appetite; for the first few days, the steroids had increased my appetite, but after that it had disappeared almost completely.

In fact, the pills messed up many of my bodily functions.

I felt so lonely and was desperate for my life not to change.

I did lots of random things; visited friends, had panic attacks with them, went walking and even worked on an organic farm.

Around that time, I started craniosacral therapy and I also scratched my entire belly, by climbing and falling out of a tree.

I went to Scotland and Spain and one day, I went for a walk in the hills near my house and fell over in some mud; I got upset about that for hours afterwards. Another time, I was by a lake in my university town with a friend, when I caught a tiny fish in some water in my cupped hands. I wondered if travelling and the sun would make me happy. I questioned finance and religion and the sleeping pills that I had completely failed to work, even when I took much more than the advised dosage; the only thing they succeeded in doing was making my eyes hurt. Later that summer, I tried to move to the Alps in France and when that failed, I very nearly got myself a mortgage on a property in the UK, because I thought that it might make me happy. I was always making plans and lists of things to do and had many different counsellors at that time.

I was desperate to feel better and often crawled in bed alongside my mum, just before she went to work. She hugged me and sometimes I felt better for an instant. Macmillan Cancer Support sent me a newsletter and I read it in bed one day. In it, I saw a picture of a man with two prosthetic legs running a marathon for the charity. I found that I was able to relate to him and the picture appealed to the fighter in me and was reminiscent of what I had been a few months earlier. I could do something like that, I thought. I was constantly dazed and quite ill, but desperate to be healthy and happy again, so I called the cancer charity to get an information pack sent to me about their up-and-coming fund-raising challenges.

After a month of being at home my parents urged me to finish my degree, so I returned to university to my room in the halls.

It was no mean feat as I was out of it most of the time and found it difficult to concentrate or even feel present during lectures. I tried to socialise with my friends, but I found that hard, too. My friend was also an insomniac and we spent one night just sitting around on sofas in her house and chatting. It was like we were at a teenagers' sleepover, minus the sleep, until dawn, that is, by which time I was exhausted and so popped a couple of sleeping pills to knock me out. I often saw Justine, Tim and Dr R, but stopped going to classes completely and avoided my classmates. My friend Jen took me to a yoga class and I enjoyed it, which was a rare feeling at that time in my life. Luckily, I only had one final exam, as my course had been modular. The exam was French translation, which I was allowed to take in a separate room to my classmates. I graduated without any academic help and gained a 2:1 degree classification; my parents watched me graduate on 14 July 2005 and it was a happy day for all concerned. I was happy for at least a few minutes that day.

Sometimes I tried jogging or rock climbing and other times I could not manage to do anything, and on one of these occasions, I wrote in my diary: I can't rock climb yet; the drugs keep making me fall over! I was my own worst enemy to try and get better around, as I didn't help myself. I was horrible to myself and always making myself do really difficult things. In April 2005, I signed up to cycle across Mexico for Macmillan Cancer Support. It was a totally impulsive decision, a complete gamble that I hoped would turn out well. I am quite an impetuous person by nature and generally very physical and I think that impulses and excessive energy can be a very potent mix. I was desperate not to be a patient of the cancer charity, but a fund-raiser for them; not a taker, but a giver. I did not like taking and would not accept that I needed to, albeit I was extremely grateful for the charity's help. I tried to convince myself that I was fine and it's one of the most stupid things that I've ever done. In the next few months, I earnestly wrote loads of letters to family, friends, businesses, rotary clubs, Women's Institutes, samba bands, radio stations, newspapers and many other organisations to try to gain sponsorship for the Mexico cycling challenge that I had committed myself to doing.

Brain surgery had left me with a three-inch scar on the back of my head; it was covered with a huge white plaster and I did my best not to disturb it. The scar was shaped like a lazy "S" and I was sort of proud of this war trophy. However, after a few weeks of not washing it, my hair got really disgusting and I decided to wash it very carefully, trying not to get any water on the scar. I did not get my hair professionally cut for well over a year, because I was scared of revealing my scar and the shaved bit of my head to anyone, as it might have prompted questions and could have potentially caused further upset for me to deal with.

Even in this weird period, I made really good friends with a girl who I rock climbed with called Jess. She was fantastic and seemed to enjoy being around me, even though I was confused about everything and frequently hated being around myself.

I continued to live in my university town for the next few months with a lady and her cat. I was seeing a guy at the time, who I'd met on a roundabout in the middle of busy traffic. On the day we met, we'd been doing a traffic survey and we both had clipboards and wore fluorescent, high-visibility jackets.

During those months, I was doing temporary administration work, jogging occasionally and kind of happy on the surface; however, my deepest upset was always lurking nearby.

Sometimes, the cat would come into my bedroom at night uninvited and curl up to sleep on my head, almost as if the animal was incubating my head, but its claws always got tangled in my hair.

I found it rather depressing when I moved back to my parents' home near Christmas time. I was doing all sorts of awful temporary administration jobs as well as training for the Mexico challenge on a bike in the cold weather and preparing for it administratively. I was totally focused on Mexico; I just wanted to be ready for the challenge. Indeed, it scared me more and more the closer it got.

5

Mexico Coast-to-Coast Cycling Challenge; El Grandisimo

Introduction for the trip by tour operators Discover Adventure Limited.

> Mexico is an enormous and varied country, with snow-capped mountains, dense jungle and cactus forests. It also has a fascinating mixture of ancient and modern cultures. Our aim is to cycle the 600 km from the Gulf of Mexico to the Pacific Ocean. The route is very hard and hot! First, we will cycle through tropical farmland, before climbing through dense jungle into cloud forest up to 3000 m, our highest point in the Sierra Madre mountain range. From there, we will cross the mountain range along small roads and potholed tracks through pine forest, until we finally descend out of the mountains to the Pacific Ocean. There are some long and very hard climbs, compensated for by some long and exciting descents. Our route will take us through many remote and small Indian villages and colonial towns. Please note, this is a tough and adventurous trip.

This cycling challenge was very hard and took place between 4 and 16 March 2006. Nothing compares to the physical and emotional pain it caused me. I was there to prove I could do it, to myself and everyone else. This was my statement to the world:

I'm OK, really I am. I can cycle across Mexico. Looking back, I can see that it was not necessarily kind to do all that to myself. It hurt so much to know that I had a brain tumour, I cannot express the magnitude of that pain in words. It was a relentless cause of distraction and anxiety for me. I have always been a very physical person, so my reaction to such huge emotional upset was logically hugely physical. So my physical success in cycling across Mexico was directly fuelled by my emotional upset. Throughout the whole ride my legs were shaky and my whole body ached. My mind was similarly all over the place. I couldn't concentrate; I didn't want to eat and I hated the thought of getting back on to my bike and what became a really uncomfortable and painful saddle. I don't know how I did it but I guess it took a great deal of superhuman determination.

Riding across Mexico was a bizarre, dazed and out-of-body experience; so much so that I was very distracted mentally and only conscious of extreme physical pain and danger. In this state, I hardly took in much of the Mexican scenery, so my descriptions of it are few. I also have few smell or taste memories of the country, a way in which I normally experience travelling. Looking back, it is hard to believe it was me that did all that, but, simultaneously, my memories of the event are extremely vivid.

Saturday 4 March 2006. Day One. 0 km cycle distance.

> Discover Adventure Itinerary: Depart UK – arrive Mexico City and transfer to our hotel on the edge of town.

On 4 March, I arrived at London Heathrow Airport at 8.00 a.m. an hour late, to meet the rest of the group and check in for my plane. Sarah, one of the event organisers from Macmillan Cancer Support, was already there and gave me my ticket for the trip; I was the last in the group to check-in. The group I was cycling with across Mexico was called Team Macmillan and was comprised of forty-two people. A few older twenty-somethings, thirty-somethings and middle-agers, I was the third youngest at twenty-three, with Nat, twenty-two, and Marco, twenty. We were all raising money for the charity for our own personal reasons. The trip was organised by Discover Adventure, our tour operators, with three of the crew cycling with the team as well as two doctors from the UK, three Mexican support vehicles, a team of three Mexican caterers and a Mexican support lorry and crew.

The plane journey was excruciatingly long; I had never flown so far before, halfway around the earth. I never got truly comfortable during the ten-hour flight and I couldn't settle down. I was sitting by the plane's kitchen, apparently a hub of transatlantic activity, the food was nasty and the in-flight films were bad. I was nervous about the bike ride and all sorts of thoughts and anxieties were racing through my mind. Could I really do it? What would happen if I couldn't? When I felt like I should have been excited at the prospect of such a challenge, in real terms I was petrified and miserable. In fact, it made me even more miserable to be thinking about it all so negatively.

I was nervous and scared of everything that day. I had never been out of any European time-zone before and yet here I was, on the plane, flying around the world towards Mexico following the sun. So that day was super-long and, in the same way that a child is scared of the dark, I was really freaked out by the seemingly eternal sunshine. "Why won't it stop?" begged something inside me. It was literally the longest day of my life.

The long flight did, however, give me the chance to meet some of my teammates on the flight, who all seemed nice.

We landed in Mexico City at around 8.00 p.m. Mexican-time, six hours behind UK time; in other words, 2.00 a.m. in my head.

My body and mind begged to relinquish consciousness and go to sleep, but by 9.00 p.m., Discover Adventure and the team were involved in a full-on bike crisis. There were not enough bikes to go round – had the airline left some behind at London

Heathrow? Yes, but I did not care at all, I just wanted to lie down on the floor of baggage reclaim, close my eyes and vanish. I was completely overwhelmed with a huge gnawing feeling in my stomach. Why was I here? The bike crisis continued and we were forced to stay in the airport for ages. I knew that someone was busy stressing about it and meanwhile, I met Nat. She had caught a different flight to meet the rest of the group in Mexico and we sat on the airport floor and got on well together from the outset. She was about my age, a student and from northern England like me, and we became great friends; a double act never to be apart on the epic adventure that was to follow. I am so glad that I was there with Nat supporting and encouraging me, as I could not have done it without her. I helped her, too, and we really leaned on each other throughout our time in Mexico. Eventually, someone resolved the bike crisis and the group piled on to the coaches beneath the stylish 1970s interior of Mexico City International Airport.

It was 11.00 p.m. and at our hotel, somewhere in Mexico City, we were allocated room and tent buddies. I was pleased to be sharing with Nat and after a plate of greasy spaghetti, the fun began. Our room was on the fourteenth floor, but none of the lifts worked. Nat had a massive suitcase and I had an equally massive rucksack and we were both shattered to the point of delirium. I don't remember the next hour clearly, but what I do know is that it involved a lot of walking, dragging extremely heavy bags up infinite flights of stairs, sneaking through a conference, trying to unlock someone else's room, and running off when the occupant came to the door and we realised our mistake. We laughed hysterically in our delirious state, laughing at this ridiculous situation in stairwells, corridors and in a briefly working lift with three Mexican boys, who must have thought we were completely high; that much was obvious by the way they glanced at each other.

Finally, we stood in our room on the fourteenth floor, with a new friend, a Mexican boy, who had kindly just carried Nat's huge suitcase up countless flights of stairs on his head and who perhaps wanted something in return. We could not speak much Spanish and he spoke no English, so, waving exaggeratedly, we repeated, 'Goodnight, goodnight,' and eventually he got the message and left. We shut the door behind him, only to find that it did not close properly, or lock, for that matter. Not at all surprised, we laughed some more and shoved Nat's huge suitcase against the door.

It was late and I hadn't got any pyjamas, I'd forgotten to bring any. I did not sleep at all that night, my head was spinning so much, and Mexico City was both hot and noisy throughout the night. This was my first night out of Europe and it felt very strange and was not at all comfortable, especially in that hotel. I suspected that gun fights and vicious killings were happening all around us and I kept waking Nat by accident, with my constant moving about. I tried to calm down by listening to the wind in the treetops on my MP3 player; it often makes me go to sleep, but the battery was running dangerously low and I knew it might die at any moment, leaving me stranded indefinitely without music or retreat.

Sunday 5 March 2006. Day Two. 0 km cycle distance.

> Discover Adventure Itinerary: After a thorough briefing, we will leave the frenetic streets of Mexico City and drive to the beginning of our ride. The journey will take around seven hours and we will pass below the smoking volcano of Popocatépetl and the highest mountain in Central America, Pico de Orizaba. We then descend through mountains to tropical farmland, eventually arriving at the coast and our starting point just south of Alvarado. We will set up camp, just south of Alvarado.

To my dismay, morning arrived all too soon and I felt as tired as I had done the night before. In a trance, I descended the fourteen flights of stairs in the hotel to eat breakfast with the rest of the team. Back in the room after breakfast, whilst packing to leave, I asked Nat why she was doing the cycling challenge and she said her aunt had had cancer. She asked why I was doing it and I replied, 'Because I've got a brain tumour and this charity helped me through it.' She stopped packing, sat down and just stared at me in utter disbelief. I had a huge lump in my throat, but desperately tried not to cry. Inside, I urged her not to stare – don't be surprised, it's not a big deal, it's okay. Eventually, I got round to saying, 'I think I told you about that in an email,' because we had been emailing each other for a few months before finally meeting up in Mexico.

'No, Emily,' she replied seriously. 'I would have remembered something like that. I guess that kind of thing either makes or breaks you.'

I hoped it would make me, but felt uncertain; besides, at least the emotional moment had passed and I had escaped crying in front of her. I was dealing with some terrifying emotions and was desperate to front it all with a brave face; indeed, this was a cruel way to treat myself.

It was sunny in Mexico City and at 8.00 a.m., the whole of Team Macmillan and the Discover Adventure crew piled on to two coaches, with all our luggage and equipment. We were heading to the east coast, to the region of Veracruz, where the pan-Mexico nightmare would begin. I was full of dread, but grateful for some respite before the challenge began. The colourful graffiti, dust, roads, buildings, cars and people of Mexico City fascinated me as we drove through and I was content to feel both intrigued and distracted. I enjoyed riding in the coach and chatted with Nat in the seat behind me, momentarily feeling safe. We drove out of the city on a busy highway, through scruffy suburbs and out into the open countryside. At a checkpoint, some Mexican men in uniforms with enormous machine guns stopped the coach, walked on and ordered us to get off. I felt so excited; it was the first time I had seen so many humans carrying such big guns. I took my bag off the coach, mindful not to trust them. We were separated into two groups according to gender and the blokes were all frisked against the coach. The girls escaped the intimate search. I wanted a photo with one of these guys or, even better, I could have posed with his little pillbox cap or huge gun. However, they all looked very stern and I elected not to get my camera out for- fear of its confiscation or my being shot.

Eventually, we were allowed back on to the bus and resumed our long journey. The scenery was amazing and we drove through lush green gorges and over mountains; everything was dusty and hot. Nat and I joked about not wanting to ride up any hills or mountains like the ones we had seen that day. Little did we know that these were mere babies compared to what we'd face together in a few days. After some time, the land flattened out and the Atlantic Ocean became visible. Our coaches arrived in a field near the coast of Veracruz soon after and the start of our challenge was nigh: a cycling trek of 600 km over mountainous terrain. Fear gripped me and pitching the tent with Nat in that sloping field took a massive effort on my part.

It was late afternoon and the three Mexican caterers rocked up in a van, cooking amazing amounts of lovely food on a camp stove. The Mexican cooks were fantastic: Maria, her husband Juán and their son Ignacio, seventeen. We all became friends, despite the huge language barrier. I just smiled at them a lot. I was just being friendly but I think Ignacio had a crush on Nat, or me, or perhaps even both of us, because he used to smile sheepishly whenever we went near him and he was always staring at us. Not only this, but his dad even asked me to marry Ignacio at the end of the ride; needless to say, I declined, telling them that I was going on to Guatemala, which was completely true.

Anyway, Nat and I were flattered about Ignacio's crush and flirted as much as we could with him in the most non-linguistic way possible.

That night, I sat on the grass and ate as my teammate Dominic told me how anxious he was about the ride. I did not tell him that I, too, was terrified, as internalising my fear seemed to be by far the easier option. I have since realised that this is not a healthy option. That night, I hoped and prayed that maybe the food would be cooked badly and I would get food poisoning and be forced to drop out the next day. I was still very jet-lagged and didn't sleep well at all that night in the sloping field, with various thoughts and doubts raging around my head like a hurricane.

Monday 6 March 2006. Day Three. 92 km cycle distance.

> Discover Adventure Itinerary: After a final look at the Gulf of Mexico, we set off on our unique challenge. We begin by cycling through swamp and sugar-cane fields, passing through lots of small villages along the route. Our first stop is at Tlacotalpan, a beautiful village along the Rio Papaloapan. We then continue on to the larger and busier town of Cosamaloapan. The small road is generally quiet, but the towns are busier and in places, a large number of sugar-cane lorries have to be avoided. After around 50 km, we have lunch. The afternoon's ride takes us through yet more small villages and tropical farmland. The route is flat and the cycling straightforward, but it is often humid and hot. Our evening's camp is near the small village of San Isidro.

Unfortunately, morning arrived all too soon for the second time, bringing no stomach ache and an impending doom.

Some of my teammates called "Good morning" as I emerged from my tent and I screamed inside, oh no, this is really happening! After queuing up in the middle of the field, we ate horrible watery cinnamon-flavoured porridge and cheese pancakes. I was not hungry in the least, but figured I should at least eat something, as this would no doubt be the start of a gruelling, energy-burning day.

The three Discover Adventure crew members started allocating bikes to everyone on the basis of their height. They were all mountain bikes, but some were red and others were yellow. Red was my favourite colour and the red ones were definitely cooler, with chunkier tyres and front suspension; the yellow ones were much more basic and so I wanted a red bike.

Nat got a red bike and then my turn came, 'Emily Parr;' I got a yellow bike. Bloody typical. Then we were all given the opportunity to enhance our bikes with little bits of additional personal cycling paraphernalia. I had brought my bar ends from the UK with me and trying to fix them to the yellow bike proved to be futile, as we were missing a vital part, so no bar ends at all for me across Mexico. Again, bloody typical.

However, we put my toe-clips on the pedals, as they are supposed to increase pedal-power; but for me, they caused a huge amount of hassle, eventually causing me to fall off my bike with embarrassing ease and frequency, nearly killing myself and Nat too, with my feet trapped in the pedals. Bloody typical. After a particularly bad incident, I told Discover Adventure crew member Dougie to take the toe-clips off my bike. I was tragically under-prepared for this challenge. A lot of Team Macmillan members were good cyclists and had brought SPD shoes and special pedals to put on their bikes and increase their speed and efficiency. I wore trainers; my training schedule had also been pitiful, with lots of riding, but largely done in the comfort and confines of my own home in England on an exercise bike in front of a television, it having been too cold to venture outside. I had reasoned pathetically that training indoors with central heating was the best way to acclimatise to the heat in Mexico. I just did not want to go out in the cold and at that moment, I doubted that it had been an entirely good decision on my part. How had I even dared to believe that my training might prepare me to cycle over mountains and through rainforests? I had not even done any basic hill-training. To be honest, riding up the little hill (0.25 km) behind my house seemed impossible and when I eventually got round to trying it, it was almost impossible and left me gasping. I was, indeed, naive and daring in my scant preparation.

As the sense of doom closed in on me, wrapping itself tightly around my throat, Discover Adventure crew member Stuart briefed the whole of Team Macmillan on the mission ahead, 'You are all about to cycle across Mexico.'

I barely listened, opting for denial. I caught one of the team doctors, deeming it best to do so before we started the ride. It was Dr G, who I plucked up the courage to ask, 'Do you know about me?' She said they did from my medical form.

Months ago, back in the UK, I had talked to Dr R about this cycling challenge and he had told me I was fine medically to do it and he even encouraged me to go for it. He wrote a letter stating that my health was fine, which I copied and forwarded to the events team at the cancer charity. This was insane and there was no medical reason not to do this ride; no food poisoning or brain tumour would save me now. I filled my CamelBak with two vital litres of water; I would need every drop of it as the Mexican heat was already killing me. So to recap the reasons why I was in no fit state to start this ride: I was heavily jet-lagged, very anxious, very dehydrated, extremely under-prepared and I really did not want to be there.

Marco warmed the team up with some muscle stretches, which he did every morning before our ride over the next few days. Lots of the team members loved it; however, I didn't like it, because it always heralded the start of a new day of hellish cycling. I joined in rarely and only grudgingly, if at all.

In due course, we were ready to go, with all our gear and tents packed into the support lorry – there was nothing to stop us. Oh shit. We wheeled our bikes to the entrance of the field and waited, the atmosphere nervously tense. I saw Nat in the pack behind me, but I couldn't get to her. Then the group moved off in a flurry of clicking gears and spinning pedals. We pulled out of the junction and on to the road, off dirt and onto tarmac. I scooted my bike the first ten metres across Mexico, having trouble sitting down on my saddle. Maybe this was a bad omen for the rest of the ride that I should have heeded. It initially felt strange to be cycling on the right-hand side of the road and whilst the eight-day ride that followed caused me an immense amount of pain, it has also given me a load of fantastic memories.

Cycling away from Veracruz, the road was fairly flat and we passed through several banana plantations. I was having trouble with my toe clips right from the start and my feet simply would not go into them, which was incredibly annoying.

Eventually, the group spaced out along the road and I cycled with Nat, or just ahead of her, or just behind her. Sometimes, the tarmac ended and we were treated to cycling along stretches of crappy, bumpy roads that were more like dirt tracks. I was cycling alone at some point, when I fell into a grass verge, because my feet were trapped in the dreaded toe clips.

A couple of my teammates came and saved me; they didn't laugh, but I would have if I had been them, as I was trapped underneath my bike and couldn't move.

I was completely shattered at the halfway point that day, where we stopped in a desolate village square for lunch. The Mexican cooks were there again serving pasta and salad; Ignacio was there in all his glory! Before eating, Nat and I trekked off to find a bush to pee behind, but there none nearby, so we pissed near a big tree, which was not in the least bit hidden from view. I am sure it must have been a fabulous spectacle for the villagers.

The team was quite understandably a source of interest to many of the Mexicans we passed along our route. It must have been a bizarre sight to see and I'm sure they must have thought we were mad, as most Mexicans would never exert themselves in that heat. Only mad dogs and Englishmen! I am neither a dog nor a man, but I admit to being both mad and English.

Many roadside spectators shouted *"Hola"* or *"Gringo"*.

Gringo is non-insulting I think and means white American, but it can apply to any person with white skin. Seeing Gringo girls cycling was especially exciting to them, because parts of Mexico are very old-fashioned and females just do not ride bikes or take part in any other sort of revolutionary thing, for that matter. We really must have seemed like a bunch of cycling aliens to some of these tiny communities.

That afternoon, I trudged along on my bike, hot, tired and dehydrated. I lost Nat and collapsed on my bike at the edge of the highway; I felt like vomiting. Dr S came to see me, 'Sunstroke,' he said, and sat with me for a while. 'Ride in the support vehicle.' It was hot and I had been doing major exercise all day. I was so tired and sitting in the front of the support vehicle, I could barely keep my eyes open; I felt completely broken. Thank goodness I could not speak Spanish, so there was no chance of silly small talk with the Mexican driver.

I was upset and said simply to Dr S, 'I was only diagnosed with a brain tumour a year ago.' In fact, this small detail never left my mind; I must have been mad.

He looked at me sincerely and replied, 'I'm sure it was really hard.'

I confessed to Discover Adventure crew member Dougie that, 'Maybe I shouldn't be here; I mean, what if I'm not strong enough psychologically?'

Dougie reassured me, 'Of course you are; I know it's hard, but you'll be fine.' Dougie was a kind Scotsman with long legs.

Unfortunately, a wasp stung him near his eye on the second day of the ride and it swelled up all putrid for a couple of days.

I had cycled 75 km of 92 km that day, the vast majority of the distance. I was annoyed to have got sunstroke and dropped out so soon and I wondered if it meant that I had failed. I closed my eyes and drank water as we drove to that night's campsite, in another field of tents. Nat met me there and asked, 'Where did you get to?' I could have replied with the same question. As I lay in the tent, the thought that this was just the beginning and the ride would go on for several more days tired me out even more. Yet I felt I had to prove something to myself and with my efforts of endurance, I knew the cancer charity would benefit significantly. Nat persuaded me to come out of the tent and I noticed that we were on a farm and looking around, we soon discovered that there were no showers, however we found a big barrel of scummy water. So we laid aside our pride and used a bucket to tip cold, scummy water over each other. It was both disgusting and refreshing!

Afterwards, we sat with some of our teammates talking and looking over a huge river. I sipped rehydration salts and talked to Robbie for the first time. Robbie was a thirty-something, with tanned skin, striking blue eyes and no hair, except for a Mohawk stripe down the centre of his head. We became really good friends from our first conversation and he, Nat and I were often together throughout the trip. Team Macmillan was so big that it was hard to get to know everyone and it naturally split into cliques both on and off the bikes. I did not get to know my teammates very well, as I was far too preoccupied with my own thoughts during the week that I spent with them. For the most part in the team's social structure, couples stayed together and people stuck with others of around the same age or cycling ability; it was just human nature. I met lots of really lovely people that week and I firmly believe that everyone on Team Macmillan was amazing, because they had all committed to raising the £2,900 minimum sponsorship and had cycled across Mexico for Macmillan Cancer Support. People were doing it for all sorts of reasons – some just loved cycling and fancied doing a huge challenge to raise funds for a great cause and others had family or friends who had suffered from cancer and were thus inspired to raise money for the charity. Everyone had a personal reason for doing the challenge and I heard many of their inspirational tales. But no reason was more personal than Robbie's or mine; we were both riding to thank the charity for helping and supporting us when we needed it most. "They helped me get here today and, thank

God, I'm still alive" and I had to constantly remind myself of this fact, when riding up those painful mountains.

I sat in the grass with Robbie later that day and I thought he might have had cancer, because I thought that he looked like he might have had chemotherapy. He told me he had been diagnosed with a cancerous tumour behind his nasal cavity three years previously and that he'd had chemotherapy to treat it. He was still recovering and looking forward to drinking a beer, because he still couldn't drink alcohol yet. He was there because he believed that the cancer charity was a fantastic cause; they had helped him through the challenge of being diagnosed with cancer by allocating him a specialist Macmillan nurse. I told him that I had a benign brain tumour and that the cancer charity had also sent me a specialist nurse. My nurse had been by my side in the doctor's office from the very first moment I had been told of my diagnosis nearly a year previously and I am incredibly grateful to him and the charity for that. I'm so glad he was with me, otherwise I would have been alone and even though it blew my head off, his constant support made the bullet somewhat easier to bite. I was so thankful that I felt prepared to cycle across Mexico and earn the charity loads of sponsorship to prove it and in the process, I had to tell everyone I knew that I had a life-threatening condition. Small price. I liked the way that Robbie stared at me after I told him. I could detect no shock or horror in his eyes, like I had seen in the reactions of other people, outsiders to this kind of thing. Instead, I felt some kind of concern and serene understanding, which made me feel calm; indeed, I found I was no longer struggling not to cry when I was with him, like I had done so often when I explained the brain tumour situation.

Someone called to announce that dinner was ready and everyone disappeared off to eat. Robbie and I remained sitting in the long grass outside his tent for a while. The air was still warm and it was a sunny evening. After a moment of silent understanding, I said, 'It's scary when it's in your head, isn't it?'

'Yeh, it's really scary,' he answered quickly.

We talked for a while about tumours and cancer, which was a huge relief, because thus far on my tumour-inspired pilgrimage, no one had spoken so openly about it or made it seem so real. Robbie was a great guy and we went to eat with the rest of the team a short while later. Chemotherapy had stolen Robbie's teeth and he could no longer eat solid food. I had no appetite, feeling very shaky and unbalanced, but I managed to force-feed myself with some noodle soup and pasta – my sensible self was aware that I would need the energy. My exhausted mind and body just wanted to rest, so back in the tent after dinner, sleep came to me fast, but was disturbed and broken by the constant crowing of cockerels. We were camping in the wild most nights in fields and other random places, with holes dug for toilets at most of the sites, which was all very challenging. It was hard to rest properly in such basic conditions.

Tuesday 7 March 2006. Day Four. 85 km cycle distance.

> Discover Adventure Itinerary: Breaking camp early, we set off towards the large town of Tuxtepec. The 25 km ride along good flat roads is great fun, if a little busy. We have a short refreshment stop in Tuxtepec, before going through the busy town together and continuing towards our lunch stop beside the Rio Papaloapan. After a relaxing swim and a good lunch, we set off towards Valle Nacional, a small town set at the foot of the mountains. The quiet road climbs gradually through low foothills and dense jungle. Camp is located near San Mateo Yetla beside the river.

I woke early at 4.00 or 5.00 a.m., because I was anxious about the day ahead. Broken sleep like this had plagued me since my hospital visit a year beforehand and it left me feeling very tired all the time. That night had been no exception for me and after lying in the tent fully awake until 6.00 a.m., Nat woke up and the day began. We rolled up our sleeping bags and mattresses and packed them away and then we transplanted our things that were strewn everywhere in the tent into my rucksack and her huge suitcase that would not even close. It was hilarious, Nat had brought a huge suitcase on wheels camping and it would not even close, because some person or other at the American customs had broken it on her journey from Manchester to Mexico. We dismantled the tent and rolled it into its bag and then rucksack, suitcase and tent were dragged across the field to the support lorry, which took all our gear on to the next campsite. There were some good-looking guys in the Mexican support lorry crew, which presented another excellent flirting opportunity. "*Gracias*", with a cheeky smile and eye contact, was pretty effective. This whole exasperating rigmarole happened every morning (except for the last one and I will explain all about that later). It exhausted me before we had even considered going near our bikes. Next, it was time to force down some breakfast on the ground outside in an open space, although I was never actually hungry.

Breakfast was muesli, cheese pancakes and fruit – what I needed was energy and a miracle escape route.

After Marco's team warm up, we were back on our bikes beginning yet another day. My toe clips thwarted me again and embarrassingly, I fell over in the dirt before we had even moved off. Day two was tough; I was still completely jet-lagged and spaced out. We rode through searing heat and I drank gallons of water, mindful not to get sunstroke again. I rode with Nat and Robbie, encouraging each other along the way and Robbie kind of adopted us and stayed with us. We ended up riding near the back of the group most of the time without any magic, speed-enhancing equipment between us. That was fine by us and the general consensus in our little group was that this was a pan-Mexico ride to be enjoyed, not a race. If it had been a race, I would not have got involved, as I dislike competition and the cycling was relentlessly hard work.

Mexico Coast-to-Coast Cycling Challenge; El Grandisimo

That day, Nat and I had stopped in a traffic jam on a bridge, when my feet once again became trapped in the dreaded toe clips. My bike fell over like a big domino with me still on it. I crashed into Nat on my left and she fell off her bike in front of a stationary bus. I apologised profusely for the potentially fatal mistake, but she was badly shaken and possibly even psychologically scarred. Later, in our camp surrounded by banana trees, I asked Discover Adventure crew member Dougie to remove the toe clips from my bike, something I should have done a lot earlier. I could not go round endangering my friends' lives with my toe clip antics any more.

After lunch that day, I was riding in a group of about ten people, when something or other went wrong on someone's bike. I forget what it was now, but it was probably something like their chain coming off or their brakes or gears failing.

Anyway, we stopped by the side of the road, the offending bike was turned over and rapid repairs began. Loads of little chattering, smiling, energetic Mexican children ran out from their houses nearby, surrounding us, shaking and slapping our hands and trying to speak to us. My limited Spanish allowed me to tell a small group of girls that I was English, my name was Emily and I was twenty-three. However, the main thing was that with a lot of smiling and hand gestures, we were communicating. This was definitely the highlight of the day for me and one of my favourite events of the entire ride.

In the campsite that night, in yet another field of tents, I could not force myself to move out of my tent, because I was so immensely tired.

Wednesday 8 March 2006. Day Five. 67 km cycle distance.

> Discover Adventure Itinerary: This is the most challenging day of the trip, with an enormous climb. We begin from an altitude of 250 m and climb to 3,000 m over a distance of 67 km. Our route takes

us through dense jungle, cooler cloud forest and, once through the cloud at 2,250 km, into pine forest and later, almost bare mountain slopes. The route is extremely steep in places, especially the first 10 km and the last 5 km, and the road surface varies from smooth tarmac to muddy dirt tracks. We pass through several very small villages, but essentially we are on our own! This is a very tough challenge for everyone and requires patience, determination and stamina. We camp 9 km from the summit in a sheltered spot.

The third day of cycling had been revered as a difficult day since the moment we had received our riding schedules in the post some months before the trip and it had been the cause of much anxiety for many people in Team Macmillan including me. The chart showing the plan of action for day five was simply 67 km of steep uphill climbs. There was no way I could feel confident about completing a task like that.

It was a gruelling, relentless day with constant sunshine through immensely huge and forested mountains. The riding was hard and the badly maintained and potholed mountain roads often wound steeply upwards.

Mexico is an amazing country; there is real financial poverty in some of the regions, but seemingly so much wealth in people's happiness and attitudes. Many Mexicans shouted "*Hola*", "*Arriva*" or "*Gringo*", when we rode past. We had ridden through towns, banana, pineapple and tobacco plantations and we had even drunk beer – Mexico is the home of popular Corona beer. Some Mexican guys would wolf-whistle at Nat and me; presumably because we were Western girls on bikes.

Whilst I was riding uphill with two teammates that day, a pickup truck full of pineapples came by and a lady leaned out of the cab and offered us a pineapple (in Spanish, of course).

We said no, and she drove off, but in the following moments we realised what it was she had offered and kicked ourselves. Then we rode past some workmen, who looked pretty intimidating, and one of them shouted *"Hola, baby"* at me. That was when I decided to give up on day five and catch a lift in a support vehicle, because I had painful stomach ache from being hunched over on the bike for hours on end under the scorching sun. I had bouts of stomach ache throughout the majority of the ride, which was uncomfortable and made my stomach feel weird. Even Robbie had to give up the ride that day, only this time it was for good; he was gutted, having waited for years for this chance to prove himself. He was having chest pains and did not think it was worth potentially endangering his health to carry on with the ride. He rode in one of the support vehicles the rest of the way, helping to man water stations at regular intervals along the route until the last day. I was sad, because I understood how badly he wanted to do this challenge and what it really meant to him. However, it only made me more determined to ride as hard as I could.

Loads of Team Macmillan cyclists gave up on the infamously gruelling day five and as Discover Adventure had planned it to be extremely tough, even they did not expect many people to finish it. However, a handful of hardcore cyclists did complete the day, much to their merit, and quite understandably, they were all completely knackered.

However unrealistic it was, I was a bit disappointed not to have completed all 67 km of day five, but I rode 30 km of it and gave it my best shot, and besides, my stomach was crippling me.

Thursday 9 March 2006. Day Six. 57 km cycle distance.

> Discover Adventure Itinerary: After the challenge of the previous day, we set off with slightly aching limbs. A downhill section to start with is a welcome relief to the previous day's climbing. After an initial descent, we climb for several kilometres through coniferous forest and then have a fantastic 20 km descent along potholed roads to the town of Guelatao, where we can

stock up on snacks and cold drinks. A further 6 km of descent takes us to our lunch stop beside Rio Grande. Our afternoon's ride is part of a long and steep 14 km climb.

Our beautiful campsite is situated around halfway up the hill.

The trip would coincide with the one-year anniversary of my brain surgery, which I thought about a lot both before and during the trip and I concluded that it would be an excellent celebration. A completely fantastic antithesis. Reality though, was such a contrast. On 9 March 2005, I had been as high as a kite on morphine after brain surgery and on 9 March 2006, I would be higher than a kite, at literally 3,000 m, cycling over mountains in Mexico.

I woke up confused and thought it was 10 March at first and that I had missed the anniversary. I was relieved that I would not have to deal with all that additional emotional shit and my confidence was boosted by the thought that I had done my one-year anniversary the previous day without even realising it.

However, later in the day, I realised that it was in fact 9 March and indeed, my anniversary. Having not finished the previous day, I was even more determined to finish this one.

It was a beautiful sunny day again and I felt so proud to be able to complete the full 57 km of day six; in fact, it was extremely satisfying, because of the extra significance for me.

The morning included lots of fun riding downhill and then the afternoon offered 14 km of steep uphill climbs in scorching heat, with no shade; it was awful, but I did it mostly on my bike, riding very slowly and staring at the road a few metres ahead of my bike for several hours. Nat and I encouraged each other all the way, as I seriously thought that I might faint from the heat.

We named ourselves Team Snail, due to our speed; sometimes, I rode slower than she could walk whilst pushing her bike. At the end of the 14 km climb, I was on autopilot, like I had been when I'd run the London Marathon; I was physically shattered, but my mind took over and somehow, I kept going. All the way up that hill I'd thought of the people I care most about and it kept me going.

I had achieved a lot that day and had battled with irritating menstrual issues, plus an upset stomach and the scorching sun.

I had to laugh, all these extra problems seemed ironic, as if the one-year anniversary of brain surgery was not enough for me to deal with. I felt like a winner having overcome all of this and just felt that life is inescapably epic.

Friday 10 March 2006. Day Seven. 75 km cycle distance.

> Discover Adventure Itinerary: Starting early, we attack the remaining 17 km of the climb. We pass through the small village of Punto and finally reach La Cumbre at 2,800 m. The view is spectacular. Below, you can see Oaxaca; a large bustling city lying on a flat, open plain, with mountains beyond. From the top, we have a great 18 km descent to the outskirts of the city, before regrouping and cycling through Oaxaca together.
>
> After a quick lunch, we continue along flat roads to the pretty town of Zaachila, where we have a short break. Leaving Zaachila on dirt tracks, we make our way up to the main Puerto Escondido road and cycle to Zimatlan, where we make camp on the edge of town.

This was a really long and gruelling day. In the morning, we did a tough uphill ride, followed by a long, fast, downhill section to the city. Nat had a hard day, so I stuck with her. We both had crazy hormones and they are not fun at any time, and especially not on a coast-to-coast cycling challenge in Mexico.

It is so important that friends stick together when they need each other. After lunch in Zaachilla in a pretty town square, with flowers covering a clock tower and with lots of people milling around, Nat called her mum back in the UK and was overwhelmed with emotion, so she cried and I hugged her. We rode away from Zaachilla on several kilometres of dirt tracks. I hated this bumpy surface, which eventually turned into a version of broken tarmac and at one point, I even threw my bike down on the side of the road, shouting and swearing angrily, all because of the road surface. I climbed down the bank into a crater of dirt to pee and I did not want to get back on my bike, but Discover Adventure crew's Jackie convinced me to shout louder about the things that were annoying me and then get back on my bike. Later in the afternoon, the whole of Team Macmillan regrouped and passed through Oaxaca as a huge fleet of cyclists – it must have been an awesome sight and certainly felt great for me to be a part of. We went the wrong way and all did a huge U-turn, stopping the bewildered Mexican traffic in the middle of a busy highway.

Oaxaca is a horrible city, stinky and busy, and I disliked riding in cities at the best of times. Out of Oaxaca, we broke into groups again along the highway. By the side of the road was a dead dog on its back with its legs sticking straight up in the air; it was surrounded by a pack of wild dogs and I rode on by quickly, but Marco decided he simply had to stop and go as close as he dared to get a photo. We rode eighteen long, boring kilometres along the highway to the campsite; the roads were all flat, with a mean headwind.

The campsite was yet another field, though with a swimming pool and a shower block this time. Emptying my whole rucksack on the ground, I then showered and washed all my clothes by hand, but the showers ran out of water. On the outside wall of the shower block was a sketchy-looking electric socket and I dared to hope that I could charge my MP3 player in it. I just wanted to hear music, my favourite form of escapism, so I was elated when the adaptor worked and my MP3 player began to charge without exploding. I slept fitfully again that night, but at least I was able to listen to some music.

I chose to lie there listening to Tommy Guerrero, my favourite new music artist at that time.

I thought of the future and of what I wanted to do when I returned to the UK. I did not want to do temporary administration work again, because I hated that job with a passion. Having just finished university, I was still very confused about what to do with myself. My thoughts often turned to the people that I missed and I desperately wished they were with me at that time to relieve the pain of this cycling challenge somehow, to ride with me and to enable them to understand what it meant to me to be there.

Saturday 11 March 2006. Day Eight. 95 km cycle distance.

> Discover Adventure Itinerary: After a good breakfast, we head out across the flat, hot plain through an intensively farmed region. The roads are good and the riding is generally fairly flat. Along the route there are several cafes offering freshly squeezed orange juice – a great thirst quencher! After 45 km of largely flat riding, we have a 9 km gradual climb before lunch.
>
> The cafe at the top offers welcome cold drinks and a good spot for lunch. After lunch, we have a 14 km descent into Sola de Vega, a small and remote town. A 17 km climb follows, through terraced farm mountain slopes and then coniferous forest. On reaching the top at 2,250 m, we have a fun 10 km descent to our campsite perched on the mountainside.

Nat and I did the 17 km climb together that afternoon, escaping the constant whining of some cyclists by riding fast uphill; it hurt, but was worth the pain, because they were so annoying. The climb was hard, but we kept on and reached our target. The road just kept going upwards in endless hairpin turns, but we got there in the end and earned mega amounts of respect from the rest of the team. What goes up must come down, so, in the afternoon, the two of us rode downhill for two hours, down endless, steep, hairpin bends. It was fast, dangerous and fun, but by the end, my hands ached, as I had not worn my cycling gloves. This was the true sign of an amateur cyclist and I never made this mistake again, because gloves really do protect your hands. Riding downhill for such a long time over rough roads, my hands had absorbed every single shock from the front tyre through the handlebars. So that's what cycling gloves are for, I realised for the first time.

Nat and I had done well all day and despite all the dangerous hairpin bends, neither of us had fallen off our bikes.

Then, ten metres before we pulled into the campsite, both of us fell off our bikes at the same time into a ditch at the side of the road. We did the only thing you can in a situation like that, we laughed. Delirious, hysterical, euphoric laughter. That night's campsite was a small lay-by beside the road and although it was cramped, we found a space in which to dump our bags and pitch our tent almost under where a support vehicle had parked by the food hut. We were still laughing furiously – so hard, in fact, that it hurt. We could not stop and it was such a good release of our pent-up emotions that it did the pair of us the power of good. We were laughing at what we had accomplished and how ridiculous it all seemed. Marco thought we were funny, two girls in fits of laughter, and he wanted a photo of us laughing, but once on camera, we immediately stopped laughing. The euphoria was over.

That night, I ate soup and collapsed from exhaustion in the tent, too tired to even contemplate socialising with my teammates. We had pitched our tent next to the campsite bin, which was being fought over all night by vicious stray dogs. I was closest to them and what with sleeping nearest to the door, I was scared they might get into the tent somehow. At one point, their growling sounded so close to my head that I jumped across the tent on to Nat, I was that terrified. Needless to say, she woke up and I retreated quickly.

Mexico Coast-to-Coast Cycling Challenge; El Grandisimo

Sunday 12 March 2006. Day Nine. 88 km cycle distance.

Discover Adventure Itinerary: We should see the Pacific Ocean today! Breaking camp, we continue our exciting descent into San Pedro, a distance of 25 km. On the horizon, we can see the last mountain we need to scale, before seeing the Pacific Ocean and the end of the challenge. From San Pedro, the road climbs steeply and the 30 km hill starts with a vengeance. We are fit now and the climb is not too exhausting. As we climb, it cools slightly and there are several cafes offering cold drinks and a chance to rest the old limbs. Arriving at the 2,050 m summit, we could have spectacular views of the ocean. From here, we descend 33 km through dense forest and later, through dense jungle, to our campsite near the Rio Colotapec, just outside San Gabriel. We have a wonderful campsite and can relax in the cool river.

This morning's descent was fast and amazing. Then, later in the morning, Nat and I managed a 30 km cycle ride up a mountain through rainforest on a secluded mountain road; it was so exhausting that I felt like giving up completely a number of times. It was hot and sunny, but when we cycled into dense cloud, it became cold and damp, due to the altitude. The team regrouped and ate lunch at the top of this climb in a rustic shed, with a dirt floor and some chickens running around. It was the home of a family, who were friendly but shy, and they were probably overwhelmed as approximately fifty gringos cycled up to their house on top of a mountain, with support vehicles in tow, to eat tons of pasta and salad – it must have seemed very bizarre indeed. However, they served us the sweetest coffee that I have ever tasted and I somehow managed to overcome the language barrier between us and asked them if I could take a photo. They were slightly perplexed by my digital camera, when I subsequently showed them the image of themselves. The camera was a gadget from a different world to theirs and it must have seemed very strange, indeed. It is always best to ask people if they mind you taking their photo first, as some people in Central America believe cameras are evil and photographs steal your soul. If you take a photo of them without asking for their permission first, they might take your camera, believing their soul to be trapped inside. I did not want that to happen to my digital camera.

We rode downhill all afternoon, the group split up and I separated off and ended up on my own, with some people ahead and others behind me. It just happened like that sometimes. I got chased by three mad dogs, one of which ran at me and tried to bite me. I was mortified and screamed, 'Fuck off!', burning away as fast as my legs would carry me. It did not matter that the dog could probably not understand my exclamation, because the main thing was that it did not bite me. The scenery was amazing as I rode through rainforest, with its huge green leaves. Further on, I stopped. Full of fear from my recent encounter with the three mad dogs, I could see that in the road ahead of me was a pack of approximately twenty animals. They looked like hyenas; hyenas in Mexico? I was so freaked out, that I turned around as fast as I could and pelted back up the hill to find a friendly teammate. When I found one, she reassured me that it was okay and we rode off together towards the hyenas. Nearing them slowly, we realised it was just a herd of goats in the road, but my teammate said we should tell everyone we had ridden through a pack of hyenas anyway, just to impress them and make the story sound a bit better. She told me one of her relatives had had cancer and died, which was why she was doing the ride with her husband. I told her my reasons for doing it and she was amazed. Again, the explanation and vocalisation of those words "brain tumour" brought a huge lump to my throat.

The campsite was by a river and we were all able to have a wash that night. The Mexican cooks served soup and food from their usual stall. The oldest member of the team told Nat and me about planes in World War II. He was bent over at the shoulders and Nat adored him, but, despite his elderly demeanour, he was an excellent cyclist and was always up near the front of the pack. The majority of the team felt excited and relaxed that tomorrow we would finally complete the challenge. Someone put a celebratory beer in my hand, but I did not want it, because I was not happy or jubilant; instead, I was tense.

This had been way more than a bike ride to me. This journey had first begun in April 2005, after I had dared to take the risk of signing up to this challenge during my enforced, steroid-fuelled illness. I had dared to be determined and believe in myself. I believed I could do this crazy challenge, wanting so badly to be fit and healthy once more, resolute in my desire to be a hero again. It was all about to end and I felt very detached. I talked to Robbie that night, explaining how I felt. Indeed, I felt empty.

Monday 13 March 2006. Day Ten. 57 km cycle distance.

> Discover Adventure Itinerary: Our final ride is a mixture of good, fast descents and several climbs, with wonderful views of the ocean ahead. As we cycle, we leave the dense jungle behind us. There is more agriculture and more habitation the closer we get to Puerto Escondido. After regrouping on the edge of town, we cycle the last 2 km together to the Pacific and a well-deserved swim! Afternoon free. Celebratory meal!

After another night of poor sleep, I woke to another sunny day. Nat and I prepared for the final day in our tent. The thought of what was happening overwhelmed me and I started to cry. Nat asked me what was wrong, but I could not explain, I was distraught, on my knees, in a tent in Mexico and I sobbed like never before. I do not remember doing this next thing, but I was in such a state that when Nat tried to comfort me, I told her sharply to, 'Fuck off!' This upset her; she felt useless and went to find Robbie to talk to me and then sat outside the tent on a rock by the river feeling like a spare part. Robbie came to see me in the tent and comforted me as tears still rolled down my cheeks; I couldn't stop them.

He said, 'I know,' and I knew that he knew something that no one else could. He knew what it felt like to be in Mexico in that field at that very moment at the end of our challenge and he understood the reason we had done it, perhaps out of a convoluted sense of duty, or maybe we were defending our pride. I looked at Nat outside the tent. 'You've upset her,' he said.

Eventually, I emerged from the tent. Some members of the team knew my reasons for doing the challenge and concern for my welfare had spread some way through the camp. Some kind teammates helped Nat put the tent down, as I was in no fit state to do it. Sarah, one of the event organisers from Macmillan Cancer Support, came to see me and we took a short walk along the riverbank. She knew why I was upset and I sobbed the now familiar, 'I was only diagnosed a year ago. I'm only twenty-three.' I felt it was all so unfair. All I could think was, I'm Emily Parr, I'm happy, I smile a lot, I'm concerned about others, I do a lot of things, I'm successful. I can't have a brain tumour; I do not have time for this to happen to me. But the overwhelming truth was that I did have a brain tumour.

Sarah replied, full of concern, 'It must've been so hard. You've got one of the most personal reasons in the group for being here.'

Eventually, I stopped crying and Sarah convinced me to eat some breakfast, but hunger eluded me once again. I force-fed myself a cheese pancake and some porridge with syrup, my pragmatic self still aware that I would need the energy. The team's star cyclist was a really nice guy, who was always up at the front of the pack, breaking his own records from previous charity rides across Mexico. When he saw me that morning, he said nothing, but just gave me a huge hug.

Mexico Coast-to-Coast Cycling Challenge; El Grandisimo

Discover Adventure crew member Stuart gave the team our customary morning briefing, saying, 'Just because it's the last day, doesn't mean it'll be easy,' he warned. 'The terrain is quite undulating and there are a few hills.'

This meant "It would be bloody hard", as the ride was always hard when Stuart said it would be "undulating". Emotions put to one side, I was now fully focused on what lay ahead.

Marco was, as ever, the centre of attention, wearing only tiny hot pants, a bow tie and cuffs to do his last team warm up. I think he knew all the ladies loved his looks and physique and was playing up for them! He did plenty of bending over to show them his cute little arse; it was all very funny. Marco kept his "outfit" on for the entire day and we laughed about it later.

I was really pleased that Robbie had decided to get back on his bike and ride on the final day. The team set off as a big group, but soon broke off into smaller groups. I rode with Nat and Robbie, but then something crazy and exciting happened inside of me. Adrenalin took over, like when I have been running and felt the so-called "flow". This is the feeling I get when my body is functioning really well. It feels incredible and so harmonious that I think I could run forever. I had experienced this feeling when running the London Marathon in April 2004. During the last mile of the marathon, I was in excruciating pain and yet I got a huge surge of energy and started sprinting, like emergency canisters of energy were firing off in my leg muscles. It was as though the pain was so great that it became white pain, so huge and omnipresent that it almost became insignificant. At that point in the marathon, it began pouring with rain. I can honestly say that I've had a few very moving moments, when I have been completely soaked with rain and running. The same thing happened that day on my bike, except this time it was very sunny. All the upset and emotional turmoil that I had felt was turned into raw energy; indeed, I was so emotionally charged that instead of feeling the huge emotions, my mind converted their pain into energy. My body just functioned on its own – I had no choice and began to pedal really hard. Right, let's just get this bastard ride finished, I said to myself. I left Nat and Robbie riding together. I did not want to leave them, but inside, I knew I simply had to speed up.

I cycled alone for a while through forest and up hills with people some way ahead and behind me. My thighs burned going up those hills, but my mind ignored the pain and I kept up a high rate of pedal revolutions. It surprised me that I could do that to myself, I was on complete autopilot; it hurt and I was enjoying it in a sadistic kind of way. I surprised even myself, as I passed people in the team who I had never seen cycling before, because they were normally at the front of the pack and I was usually at the back partying with Nat and revelling in Team Snail. I kept going and rode fast and furiously and soon, I was on my own again and cycling down a very long, straight and dusty highway. There were few cars on the road that day and cycling along the highway, I realised that I had been alone for a very long time and wondered if somehow I had gone the wrong way. But I could not have, as there had been no major junctions for me to have taken the wrong direction at. So I continued on my own, slightly nervous and hoping to meet the others in the team later. I ran out of water and stopped twice to buy drinks; it was extremely hot and I needed fluid. I enjoyed talking to the shopkeepers in my limited Spanish and the best shop I entered was like a living room with a sofa. It was run by two little girls of about ten and eight years old and they got me a Coke, even though I had requested Pepsi. They talked to me and I told them my name, my age and where I was from and with plenty of hand gestures and smiles, we understood each other quite adequately enough. I filled my CamelBak with Coke and rode on.

Eventually, I came to a major fork in the highway and just as I was thinking, oh no, which way now? I heard cheering and clapping and saw some of the team members at a cafe in the middle of the fork. I felt relieved to see them and they were cheering for me! I rode over to them and got off my bike.

Mexico Coast-to-Coast Cycling Challenge; El Grandisimo

Someone hugged me, 'Nice one, Emily,' they were surprised that I had finished so early. That was it, the suburbs of the final destination, Puerto Escondido. I had cycled across Mexico from the Atlantic to the Pacific! But I still had to see the ocean to believe it. I heaved an enormous sigh of relief, collapsed on to the pavement and melted. The team was regrouping at this cafe, before riding together to the sea in a huge fleet. It was monumental and I talked excitedly with my teammates. We cheered noisily for all the others who rode up to the cafe, each one was a hero. About ten or fifteen minutes later, Robbie and Nat cycled towards us and I cheered extra loudly. I hugged them both and gave Robbie a massive kiss on the cheek; I was so proud and grateful to him for staying with Nat that morning.

'Where did you get to?' asked Nat, in a slightly annoyed tone. Then she added, without any trace of annoyance, 'Robbie said you had to go; it was something you had to do for yourself.'

And he was right, I did need to burn off into the distance and be alone that day and I felt great because of it. But I wanted to finish this epic ride with Nat and Robbie by my side, because there was no doubt in my mind how instrumental they were in getting me across Mexico, with all their endless encouragement and kind words. After ice creams, drinks, resting on the pavement and excited banter, we got back on our bikes and rode as a proud team down a hill and through the busy town. We parked our bikes outside a hotel and ran into the Pacific Ocean. This was it, this was the end I had dreamed of and the moment was tinged with both magic and sadness.

6

My Lesson Learned

I'm very proud that I raised thousands of pounds for Macmillan Cancer Support through sponsorship of my coast-to-coast cycling efforts in Mexico. However, this does not cover the cost of what they gave me, because that is priceless.

To know someone cares is priceless. Thank you so much to my Macmillan nurse Tim – thank you a thousand million times.

I could never really express in words the enormity of my gratitude to Tim and Macmillan Cancer Support.

The upset that this chunk of my life caused me did not just stop when I finished the bike ride and ran into the Pacific Ocean in Mexico; it worked something out of my system, but was just a stage in the process of emotional turmoil that I have to go through. I suspect that life is all about emotional ups and downs, but if I just tried to be happy all the time, that would be false and I'm sure that I would miss out on experiencing so much of the good stuff in life, of which there is plenty.

I have learned a lot of things through this whole experience.

I have learned how life could be stripped of everything I recognised, which is when I felt at my most vulnerable and was when I really saw what I'm made of. All human beings have the capacity to choose their attitude in any circumstance; we can all choose our own way in life. As the saying goes, "The sky's the limit". I believe that there might be a meaning in all of the suffering, beauty and chaos of this world and I choose to try and work out the message it is sending me. This is because I think there might be a Greater Plan, which is responsible for all the stuff that happens in our world. However, there may not be, in any case each individual must be responsible for their own attitude and their own actions, not expecting life to endlessly provide support and always to generate happiness, as expectation breeds disappointment.

Instead, I try to give what I can to life, take what I feel I need from it and expect ups and downs along the way.

I learned that asking "Why me?" in despair is futile when you are suffering. I took this attitude to begin with and it only seems natural to do that. I was so angry and felt it was all extremely unfair. Why me? Why me? Why me? I'm a victim.

Curiosity is always important, as was recognising that I was merely a victim and that I could not stop the situation from existing. However, I now feel that this is a silly attitude to prolong. I believe that when it's dragged out, the I-am-a-victim attitude embraces fear and brings negativity. In addition to this, wishing intensely that my life would not change was silly. It didn't change; I just had to accept that difficult experiences are a major part of life. Every single shred of fear and every huge achievement that happened was a part of my life. It seems that suffering can happen to anyone at any age; life is indiscriminate of age, if it has something to teach a person. I believe that life might be teaching us enriching information through suffering. Although it was hard for me to see a way through it, when the pain was everywhere, I think that suffering holds many lessons for those in pain, if they are prepared to learn from the experience. So I believe that somehow, suffering was a great privilege for me when I eventually allowed it to be. The lessons learned through suffering can be a source of great strength for sufferers and the people around them, who take heed of them. For example, this experience has given me a huge insight into suffering and as a result, I feel a much more compassionate human being, with a greater capacity to try and understand some of other people's suffering and emotions. I know that my experience has also taught some of the people around me a lot about suffering and given them strength as a result. I have learned not to let myself get too busy trying to control things, to let go of the less important things and to try to relax into life's rhythms.

I have learned a lot about people and human nature.

My friends' reactions were varied – some friends were wonderful and I felt I could count on them to support me and they did this by talking to me, checking up on me, cooking for me and letting me sleep in their beds when I felt awful. Other friends did not seem that helpful; I thought that maybe they genuinely didn't care. However, I must admit that I didn't communicate the true extent of my upset to my friends and family effectively, thus they couldn't react how I wanted them to, thus I had tripped myself up harshly, leaving me feeling even more upset. My stubborn nature and pride prevented me from letting them know how much it hurt. I tried to protect myself from the true horror of what was happening by internalising my feelings, but it only made me feel worse, as all the emotions remained with me, instead of unburdening myself. Some people who I hardly knew became some of the strongest people in my support network. They showed me they really cared and I am grateful to them for that. It seems that the greatest resource and strength that I, and perhaps other humans, need to survive a harrowing experience might be the knowledge that people around them do care. The real heroes are the people who care.

The book *Between a Rock and a Hard Place* by Aron Ralston is one of my favourites. On the final page, he speaks of "Cutting out something and leaving it in your past. Saying farewell is also a bold and powerful beginning". A rock once trapped him for days and he glimpsed the face of death and was forced to amputate his own arm in order to survive. I was forced to seriously contemplate a lot of things like illness and death in my own adventure and it seems that fear of the unknown dictates the general belief that illness and death are dark and ugly things, though they may be beautiful and dazzlingly bright. I think it depends on how we choose to view these issues and to live our lives. I have chosen to lose certain preconceptions in order to carry on living life to the full, keeping in mind what it means to be healthy, what it is to be challenged and how strong I am. I have learned that I, like other human beings, am far stronger than I could ever possibly have imagined. I really think we are all so capable of being much stronger than we think we are. For example, I thought training for and running a marathon tested me to my physical and emotional limits, but that was a minor event compared to what I experienced when the human spirit inside me was really challenged. I think that maybe there really are no limits where the human spirit is concerned. Being diagnosed with a brain tumour is very difficult, but it presented me with the opportunity to experience everything that happened in this story and even the bizarre opportunity to write this book. I think that opportunities must be seized, however strange they may seem, and a journey into the unknown is one such great adventure, as it seems to be the things that we have to fight for most that give meaning to life.

The night before writing this, I had an unusually scary but very symbolic and empowering dream. I dreamt that a man held a gun to the crown of my head and pulled the trigger. The shot blew half my brains out, but I was still alive. I felt awful and half dead and begged for him to kill me properly, in much the same way I'd felt about the brain tumour on several occasions.

He tried his best to kill me, shooting me many times in the body and head, but I refused to die. Then I woke up, scared but definitely alive. The message seems to be that even when tested to the limit, my spirit can never be killed. Accepting that I had something weird in my brain was hard, but everyone is unique and I know that when the human spirit is strong, nothing can touch it.

7

Back To Life

This is a surprise chapter, surprisingly good. It is six years after the original publication of this book without this chapter and my story has progressed in a positive way that I want to share with you. So my kind publishers have allowed me to add this chapter to my original text. I am 31 years old; nine years have passed since my brain tumour diagnosis when I was 22 years old. In those nine years, I've been to a lot of places, done a lot and learned a lot. I've grown up a bit and I'm a different person so I wouldn't be shocked to find that the tone of my writing has changed somewhat.

However the past nine years have been filled with my struggle to come to terms with the reality of my health condition. The original book ends on an emphatically positive note and in an ideal world I would have felt like that for good, but my situation proved to be just too overwhelming. I didn't manage to accept it and those years were very hard. I was hammered with anxiety and depression. I was still denying the impact of the brain tumour within my physical self.

Then in my mid twenties things got worse. Many of my physical capacities deteriorated including my eyesight, hearing, the functioning of my left leg, the coordination in my right hand and my balance and general coordination. All of this happened at the same time and all of it was due to the brain tumour. Deep down I must have suspected what was causing the problems but I denied it so incredibly intensely to myself that I couldn't explain it. In my fantasy mind, I was a very healthy person, so why should

I be experiencing problems like these? I was absolutely terrified. I thought I was going properly mad.

Since 2005 I had been so focused on the brain tumour not growing or my needing a 'scary' treatment like radiotherapy. It's as if I'd held my breath and wished for the world around me to stop. I didn't care about anything else but in reality the world is constantly moving and changing; it doesn't stop. At about age 30.5, after with-holding the information from medical professionals for years in an attempt to stop any 'scary' treatment being considered or going ahead, I eventually wrote a long letter to my GP (Dr T) about the physical problems I had first experienced in my mid twenties. I have to thank my mum hugely for urging and convincing me to write that letter. I was at the end of my tether by then. I needed to try a new approach. Denial just wasn't working out for me.

Dr T sent my very honest letter on to my oncology consultant (Dr A) and it started a domino-effect of tests and medical discussions. Dr A said the tumour had not grown but its presence was causing pressure on some of my important nerves, hence the physical problems I had been experiencing since my mid twenties. Dr A decided that it would be best for me to undergo a course of radiotherapy to limit further physical impairment and perhaps even improve the physical problems I was already experiencing by releasing pressure on the affected nerves. I shat myself and the part of me who had clung to denial since 2005 was disgusted that my honest letter written to Dr T had ultimately brought this upon me. However another much more optimistic part of me had awakened. This me had always been within myself but had been asleep or had somehow slipped off my radar for nine years. This me said I should give it a shot, feeling that I needed the treatment in order for the anxiety about it (that had been with me for nine years) to finally go. Like feeling nauseous but not wanting to vomit, then vomiting and feeling better than you previously imagined possible. So I decided to go with the optimistic me and sign on the dotted line saying Yes Please I Want Radiotherapy. Dr A's pen was terrible, my signature was really bad. He laughed.

What follows is a diary of my radiotherapy treatment that I wrote to my friends and family online. I made this diary to tell multiple people stuff about myself as I always seem to forget someone who deserves to know and it definitely made my radiotherapy ranting easier!

August 2 2014

For those who don't know (because I forgot to tell you, hence the creation of this online diary) this summer I'm getting six weeks of radiotherapy. It was supposed to start on July 30 but the Drs delayed it because my treatment plan wasn't ready. New start date probably Wed 6 Aug but only if the hospital ring me on Monday to confirm it.

Radiotherapy to the brain requires the patient to wear a full facial mask. It gets moulded in the fitting (Orfit) process. That means mine is the exact shape of my face. At first it is a bit of plastic that looks like a tennis racket, then they heat it up in a bain-marie-type-thing, then they put it on your face and it's pretty warm and lovely and then they mould it because it gets soft like warm wax. It gets hard when it cools down; it also shrinks a bit when it cools so it becomes uber-uber-tight. During treatment it is screwed down to a headboard to decrease movement to a max of 3mm. It is ok to wear, I don't find it scary, it is made from a grill of plastic and breathing is no problem. You can't open your eyes or mouth. I talk to nurses through my teeth. Like a robot. Just think I used to be a full-on claustrophobic. What a liberty that was.

I get to keep the mask after it's all over!

Monday August 4 2014

So it's confirmed. My new radiotherapy start date is Wednesday August 6 at 1318 hours. I called the hospital to confirm that, they didn't call me. But it is fairly early in the day so they might have rung me later. Still they can have a flying punch!

Having not seen some of you for a while, it seems kind to share my thoughts with you. This treatment does seem necessary to me.

My tumour has been present in my brain since birth or a very young age, don't know which, it doesn't even matter. It's quite possibly due to head trauma which was the very first event in my life after getting born, bad bad bad luck. Or maybe it's in my genetic bla bla. In fact it's a brain disease that you've got far more chance of winning the lottery than ever picking up. That makes me pretty rare. The tumour has followed a fairly textbook progression – not bothering me in younger years and only starting to become obvious in my teens (with my hearing problems) and twenties (with masses of deterioration of my hearing, eyesight, balance, coordination, left leg function, right hand function. I can't even run now – bummer).

Of course I'm a bit scared of the treatment but my general overriding feeling is excitement because I reckon the radiotherapy could improve my quality of life drastically.

Wednesday August 6 2014

Hey thanks for all the support. I am pretty calm about it, hard to believe I know! Emily, 'fraid you bore the brunt of the tears a few weeks ago and Sally got a good share of it too in more of a huge tantrum format, sorry guys!

Nice concise message as far as today goes: it's gonna be fine.

Treatment 1/30
I said it'd be fine and it was. I brave faced it all the way – what a trooper. I feel pretty tired now. And dizzy. Normal. I came out

of hospital with a grid mark on my face because the mask was so tight. But the next 6 weeks will be fine, bring it all on!

Later that evening: I've got a bit of a headache now but that's no surprise! I GOT NUKED. Generally I'm feeling pretty good.

Thursday August 7 2014

Treatment 2/30

Not feeling so loopy and tired as after treatment 1. Everything is good. I gave the radiotherapy team cakes and told them it was unashamed sucking up! They liked it. I'll try and film one of my treatments, the nuker-machine is pretty cool with a massive robotic arm that moves around me and zaps me from all angles. I'd like to see too, I never see anything inside my mask.

Friday August 8 2014

Treatment 3/30

All went fine. Yeh it's Friday! No more nuking until Monday. And this weekend I'm looking forward to a visit from my sis and nephew.

After today's treatment, slightly dazed and loopy, I asked the radiographers, 'So when does my brain tumour start reacting to this treatment?' I add (totally unnecessarily and hilariously), 'You know, when's it going Oh F*** They're Onto Me?' Radiographers giggle, reply, 'After the 1st treatment.' I leave thinking 'Goodness me, Parr, did you really just say that to health professionals, really? Like really really?'

Saturday August 9 2014

To be honest, I'm finding it quite challenging to drink 4 litres of squash every day and also to sleep.

Monday August 11 2014

Treatment 4/30 – 2nd week!

Treatment was fine. Bit of a headache but nothing a litre or 2 of squash won't extinguish.

    Question: (Me) 'Are the walls of this room lined with lead?' (Radiographer) 'Yes.' (Me) 'Is that to protect you radiographers from the megavoltage x-rays used in treatment because they're so dangerous?' Megavoltage x-rays are 100 times the strength of normal x-rays and the radiographers leave me alone in the treatment room before the radiation starts. (Radiographer says) 'Yes, that's why we have a maze of lead-lined corridors leading to the treatment room too.' (Me) 'Well why is it ok for me to be in here exposed to all that dangerous radiation?' (Radiographer looks a bit confused and answers), 'Because you need it.' There's something for me not to think too much about.

Tuesday August 12 2014

Treatment 5/30

Not a great day, it's been super difficult. Treatment happened fine but I've picked up a bug (sore throat, massive headache). Had it yesterday a bit but it had the decency not to be epic and full-on then. So I've added painkillers to my list of meds. Yeah more chemicals in my body!!!

    Question: (Me) 'How much does this big machine cost?' (Radiographer) 'About £2million but the lead-lined bunker we're in costs £8million to make so you're looking at £10million for the whole set-up.'

Wednesday 13th August 2014

Treatment 6/30

Treatment fine, I can't imagine ever saying anything else really. I have a treatment strategy. I just go in the room and lie really still, get the mask on and it's over in about 8/9 minutes. Some people panic in the mask because they feel trapped but I try and stay calm, focus on my breathing. I even try and smile a bit in the mask though I can move my face very little, I know it sounds nuts but it's a case of monkey-see-monkey-do, meaning if you act happy and relaxed then you might trick part of you into thinking that you are. It's psychology. It works for me.

Question: (Me) 'The mask is unpleasant but as a grownup I can handle it as a necessity. But how do you treat children. They'd freak out in a mask, surely?' (Radiographer) 'Anaesthetic. We have to knock them out sometimes (especially babies) or some children are ok in a mask and actually handle it far better than adults.'

Thursday August 14 2014

Treatment 7/30

Treatment 7. Fine. Breathe in CALM, breathe out SOLID.

Have been moved to another machine worth just over £1million, I miss the £2million baby. This new one can deliver me the same quality of treatment but it's just not as smooth and awesome.

Question: (Me) 'Why do you turn the lights off to position my head?' (Radiographer) 'So we can line up these laser beam crosses on your head mask.' (They called it a shell.)

Friday August 15 2014

Treatment 8/30

It's FRIDAY! No more nuking until Monday. Too tired today to ask questions or do fancy breathing tricks in my mask. I just lay there and I nearly went to sleep.

Sunday August 17 2014

Hi, just a shorty Sunday message. Thanks for all your support and for saying I'm being very positive etc. – that's kind. I am pretty upbeat (I really thought I'd be falling apart by now) but good things are occurring. 1. The Drs thought I might have terrible nausea all the time by now as a side-effect and I haven't had even one tiny bit (probs as I'm very healthy in general or maybe because I drink so much squash! No really! Or maybe my anti-sickness pills are just working!) 2. I can tell after 8 treatments that the functioning of my left leg is a bit better!!!!! These are 2 massive things, how can I not be happy?

Monday August 18 2014

Treatment 9/30

All fine, though every time I go to the treatment room my heart is banging in my chest! For once they played decent music – Ella Fitzgerald and Louis Armstrong singing Gershwin's 'Summertime'. Svelte jazz. None of this Avril Lavigne/James Blunt rubbish that hurts my feelings.

I wore my guardian angel necklace from a friend to treatment today for the first time and I felt incredibly safe!!

Question dialogue: (Me) 'Where will I lose hair in about 2 weeks?' (Radiographer) 'Round the back and a couple of patches near your ears, maybe, and maybe you won't even be affected by that.' (Me) 'Ok, it's not like I care loads about my hair, I just want to know if I'll be bald.' (Radiographer) 'I get it.' (Me) 'Thanks, bye.'

Tuesday August 19 2014

Treatment 10/30

Treatment went fine. Today is a good day because I'M A THIRD OF THE WAY THROUGH MY RADIOTHERAPY! To mark that occasion in the medical world I got some extra x-rays done to check all is going well.

I gave the radiotherapy team a big bag of Jelly Babies and tonight I shall award myself a chicken kebab (with garlic yoghurt sauce and chips). Then this evening I shall practise with my ukulele band. Ah yes, it's important to keep doing your normal activities to keep you sane!

Wednesday August 20 2014

Treatment 11/30

Treatment went fine today; they had some old crooner ballad on in the background.

The psychological benefit of my fantastic kebab last night is undeniable however it wasn't so great biologically; it must have been rammed with MSG and salt because I slept so badly and I was thirsty all night. Today I feel like a zombie.

Questions:

1. (Me) 'If you treat a patient whose tumour is in, for example, their torso – how do you keep them still? Do you use a torso restraint thing?' (Radiographer) 'No we just ask them to stay really still.' (Me thinking out loud) 'But what if they move a tiny bit?' (Radiographer) 'We have treatment margins.' (Me thinking) Sounds pretty dodgy to me (Me out loud) 'How much will my mask allow me to move?' (Radiographer) 'Not at all.' (Me) 'I love my mask.' (It's a love/hate thing.)

2. (Me) 'What are good things people do with their masks after treatment?' (Because we get to keep them.) (Radiographer) 'Art, craft, some people make them into hanging baskets, some people fill them with fairy lights.'

Thursday August 21 2014

At the moment I have a very crazy appetite – thank you, steroids! It's a bucking-bronco wild ride and I can go from fine to ravenous in seemingly seconds. All I can do is have healthy food ready to eat when I need it. So at 8.50 am I cooked a massive bowl of pasta with peppers, sweet corn, chick peas, kidney beans, spinach, watercress, rocket, red pesto and cheese. Just so I'm ready! I'm proud.

Treatment 12/30.

All went fine. I think I will go out on a limb and say that since I was diagnosed with this lovely brain defect aged 22, this is the best experience of my life (this statement is explained towards the end of the chapter). It definitely beats cycling across Mexico (which I did aged 23) and publishing a book (which I did first aged 25).

Since I was 22, I have dreaded radiotherapy as one of the worst experiences of my life and actually it's fine. As my psychological therapist said to me the other day: 'What does that teach you then, Emily?' Answer: 'It's stupid to be scared of stuff you know nothing about and in my case waste about 9 years being terrified for no reason.'

I had no confidence in how I'd deal with radiotherapy and actually I'm managing really rather well (massive self-praise, bugle fanfare, cheering crowds, me on a royal balcony etc.). I should have taken advice from the last chapter of my own book (written aged 24. Interesting fact: I have resisted owning a copy of that book ever because I've kind of hated it but I've tracked down a copy at my parents'). In the last chapter I say 'All human beings have the capacity to choose their own attitude in any circumstance', 'The sky's the limit', 'I think that maybe there really are no limits as far as the human spirit is concerned'.

I don't want to come across twee saying this radiotherapy is the best experience of my life in recent years. It is an incredibly challenging experience and I'm not on any extraordinary drugs to make it all seem wonderful!

To name a few of the challenges – some of the meds I take make my metabolism work in fast-forward whilst others make my guts work in slow motion. Hard to know what your body wants. My hair has started moulting loads, is it trying to fall out? Yes. I am super-tired all the time but able to shimmy round the house cooking, cleaning, watching TV etc. Radiotherapy is expected to cause temporary swelling in my brain which could cause me to become temporarily deaf or partially-sighted or it could do countless other things to me physically. But I expected many of these side-effects and Que Sera, seriously, I'll deal with it

I once asked my friend who lives in Toronto, 'Why do you love Toronto? It's a big, ugly city.' She just said, 'Because it's mine.' That's how I feel about this radiotherapy experience. I love it because it's mine and I'm acing it! That's why it's the best experience of my life in recent years.

Friday August 22 2014

Treatment 13/30

The best treatment so far because they played Dire Straits. I was grinning in my mask like a deranged chimp.

Now I get 3 days off treatment thanks to Bank Holiday Mon. I'm looking forward to visits from my 3 siblings, my twin bro's girlfriend and my 2 rascal nephews.

Question: (Me) 'I'm drinking about 4 litres of fluid a day and I'm peeing quite a lot but not like 4 litres a day, so what's happening to the rest of the fluid?' (Radiographer) 'Your body's absorbing it.' (Me) 'Is it because my metabolism has gone nuts?' (Radiographer) 'Yes.'

Tuesday August 26 2014

Treatment 14/30

Today I was bumped up to Linac 4 (nuker-machine worth about £2million) as opposed to the normal Linac 1 (worth just over £1million). I told the radiotherapy team I felt like I'd come home.

I showed them my hair loss (which is around the base of my skull at the back) and asked if more would fall out. They couldn't say as everyone is different. They said I could get a free wig; they always say that and I always cringe inside.

However on the way home I reconsidered; if I am entitled to a free high-quality wig then I should peruse the options. I could get a great pink, blue or glittery party wig! Is it dodgy of me to think that way?

My bald head patches feel nice. You know how nice it feels when you've shaved your legs? Well transfer that feeling to your head. IMMENSE. Came home from hospital and got my ma to rub E45 into my bald head bits because I have to moisturise them loads.

Anyway the best part of today was definitely going swimming with my genius nephew. He is nearly 2 and already has great floating skills! Today in the pool I tested my silicone swimming hat. It's brill. Head/hair/ears stayed totally dry. MAJOR BREAKTHROUGH as I love swimming!

Wednesday August 27 2014

Treatment 15/30. HALFWAY POINT

Treatment was fine today, treatment music: easy listening funk (raised eyebrow). So halfway, I've summitted, topped out. This is the top, now it's all downhill, I hope. From doing ridiculously long runs in the past, I know that the first half is always the hardest psychologically because in the 2nd half every step you take is taking you home!

I took the radiotherapy team some chocolate and sweets as a halfway present. I said I'd considered getting them a healthy gift but one of them said Who Wants To Be Healthy? I agree when it comes to chocolate and sweets ONLY.

Question: (Me) 'What do you do when the door beeps and you leave the room?' (Radiographers) 'Come and see.' (Me) 'Ok.' (We go into their office where I can see six computer screens. They explain the complex stuff they do) Bla bla bla (me) 'Ok, that's sounds complicated, so you don't just press GO and have a cup of tea?' (Radiographers) 'No.'

Thursday August 28 2014

Treatment 16/30

Again, treatment fine. Cruise control.

Question: (Me) 'All you radiographers are pretty young, any reason for that?' (Blonde Radiographer) 'No reason.' (Me) 'Well I can't really tell people's ages because I look about 3 and I'm 31.' (Brunette Radiographer) 'I'm 26.' (Blonde Radiographer) 'I'm 21, I'm the baby of the team!' (I had my treatment, 8/9 mins zapping, then they let me out of the mask. Immediately I said) 'I can't believe you're 21, I mean how have you finished uni?' (Blonde Radiographer) 'I did on the job training. I get my results next week.' (Me) 'Well I think you should definitely pass and I'm a patient so my opinion should count, right?' (The Blonde Radiographer got a well deserved Distinction in her results).

Friday August 29 2014

Treatment 17/30

Wow we're really getting on with this treatment stuff. I mean 17/30 sounds like a big deal. I'm a fair way through it.

I realised maybe I'm not painting you a realistic picture of radiotherapy treatment by saying it's all fine etc., maybe it seems easy peasy. It's not a challenge-less situation. Let me name a few of the 'negative' things that happen all the time that I could go on about: sometimes bloody gunk comes out of my ears and nose but the Drs reckon that's normal, I'm easily exhausted, I get constant headaches, my life is a meds riot, my digestive system has gone wild. Sometimes when something is wrong with me I get emotional and then I have to work out the problem; it's not always obvious. First I eat some stuff in case I've got secretly hungry then I take paracetamol in case I'm actually in pain. It's true, I can't always feel hunger or pain.

However I have chosen not to go on about all these little tedious things because IN MY MIND RADIOTHERAPY IS FINE! There we go, that's what I think the most important factor is. Your attitude, how you choose to position your mind.

In the months leading up to the treatment, my imagination got a bit crazy (mind not well positioned at all). I knew radiotherapy was coming but not what it would do to me. Dr A was legally obliged to tell me the awful truths that in very rare cases radiotherapy can paralyse or kill patients. It freaked me out. So in comparison to feeling like that, yes I think radiotherapy is fine.

My buddy took me to hospital today, we had so much fun! She had a great educational trip and the radiography team were very welcoming to her, letting her in the treatment room when my mask was put on and watching the whole treatment process in the radiography office. The radiographers made her part of the team for the day so maybe I should call her Emily Radiographer? She seemed suitably impressed by it all!

Afterwards we went to a café for tea, hot choccy and a sausage sandwich!

Monday September 1 2014

Treatment 18/30

Back to it, the daily grind. It's the first day of autumn – Oh well, sigh. So far it has been possible for me to wear shorts to every single one of my treatments but I may have to stop that if it gets cold. Or I may just wear shorts anyway in a stubborn protest.

Radiotherapy has succeeded in making me very tired; that's supposed to happen. The wig hunt is off, I can't be bothered, I'm too tired and anyway deep down in my heart I know it's not fair to raid the NHS' resources just so that I can have a free party wig.

Today in treatment the mask was so tight that most of my face went numb and my jawbone ached. What can be done about this? Well I just tried to relax my face a bit more and also to ignore it. It helped. I could have flapped my arms around and made the radiographers come and set me free but that would've been pointless – I would've just ended up back in the mask anyway having wasted some time.

To pass the time, I have been sewing a patchwork playmat for my friend's baby and tomorrow I will go on my first cookery course, ooh!

Tuesday September 2 2014

Treatment 19/30

Exciting day. Treatment fine, more than fine, very fine. Jaw-achingly tight mask again but very interesting music choices: song 1. 'A Whole New World' from Aladdin, I love it in a cheese-fest kinda way; song 2. 'All By Myself' by Celine Dion. The irony of song 2 made me grin. This is not the best song to play to a person in a 100% head restraint with 0% vision; the point is it would be easy to feel alone in that situation anyway!

Question: (Me) 'My mate works on the children's ward here. She's a puppet therapist and storyteller. I've got one of her puppets here (Benny the gnome), would you mind taking a photo of me in my mask with Benny and Cuddles the teddy bear to show kids that it is ok to have radiotherapy?' The radiographers were really happy to help. At the end they all piled in the room to get a photo of more people.

Wednesday September 3 2014

Treatment 20/30, two-thirds of the way through.

Now I can start THE FINAL COUNTDOWN: 10 to go

There will be no kebab celebration tonight; I've matured since those days (2 weeks ago). I know the MSG will unsettle me. I'm wise to it now.

Had a little treatment review with Dr A today. Short and sweet. (Dr A) 'How are you?' (Me) 'No complaints so OK I think' (Dr A) 'I'll reduce your steroids in 10 days. Remember not to expect any major changes until a few weeks after treatment when the nerve inflammation has reduced.'

Music of the day: a rare acoustic version of 'Mr Brightside' by The Killers. This song reminds me of my trip to Canada, particularly the time I spent in Banff (where the chipmunks are fat and friendly because tourists feed them too much). So I went off on a mind-holiday in my mask and ended up at Lake Louise, Canada where the water is bright blue because the water is glacial, it's stunning.

Thursday September 4 2014

Treatment 21/30. FINAL COUNTDOWN: 9 to go

Treatment went absolutely fine. No music today.

Went swimming before treatment and silicone swimming hat FAILED. Head got a bit wet, I dried it but I thought the radiographers might tell me off. They didn't.

Question: (scraping the question barrel perhaps? Me) 'What if we lived on a fault line like in LA and we had a high risk of earthquakes. What if one happened when I/another patient was stuck in their mask?' (Radiographer, complete with slightly confused face) 'Well there'd be a contingency plan like we have in case there's a fire and we have to get out of here.' (Me) 'So you wouldn't just run off without setting your patient free?' (Radiographer) 'Definitely not.'

Friday September 5 2014

Treatment 22/30. FINAL COUNTDOWN: 8 to go

Treatment went tickety-boo today. Mum came and had a scope around and concluded that it's amazing.

It's acting like autumn today but I'm still wearing shorts. I got hold of a Mint Cornetto after our visit to hospital. I have wanted one all summer but they were sold out everywhere. The ice-cream helps to soothe my mouth as radiotherapy makes it a bit sore. Maybe now I've had my Mint Cornetto I will be able to accept the coming of autumn with more grace?

Sunday September 7 2014

Didn't swim yesterday because I picked up a stomach bug. I can't blame it on radiotherapy because the treatment is very localised meaning it's only supposed to do stuff to my brain and not compromise the rest of me at all.

Wanted to explain something bizarre to you. It's about these weird sounds I hear sometimes; they're loud enough to keep me awake sometimes. The sounds are in my head physically but not in my imagination. I hear noises like the eerie creaking movement of a glacier as it flows downhill. I think this is called White Thunder. Or it could be compared to the noise of boulders being dragged along the bed of a fast-flowing river and smashing into each other.

This stuff doesn't hurt me at all, I just assume there's some kind of reorganisation going on in there. The Drs say it's normal. Normal? Er getting sugar on your face when you eat a jam doughnut is normal. Such noises seem fairly abnormal to have in your head!

Monday September 8 2014

Treatment 23/30. FINAL COUNTDOWN: 7 to go

Treatment fine. Mum showed up in the room when they took my mask off. Surprise!

Today I did an experiment. I thought radiotherapy masks were meant to impede head movement 100%. These crazy-tight masks do the best job possible BUT THEY CAN'T SUCCEED 100% as there is soft tissue attached to your skull so you can wiggle a bit (like skin and muscle). Anyone can do this experiment, you don't need a full facial mask. To understand what I'm on about, press the palm of either hand flat against your forehead, press hard then see if you can move your hand from left to right. You can. I told the radiographer who said it was accounted for with treatment margins. Alarming, I feel.

Today it is sunny and warm, I'm still wearing shorts. I think I'll manage to wear shorts to all of my treatments. It feels more summery again. I think I'll take Mum's advice and hold out for another Mint Cornetto before I let it be autumn!

Went and hoovered in my grandparents' house after hospital as I just wanted to do something useful, out of my house, having spent all weekend being ill in my house.

Tuesday September 9 2014

Treatment 24/30. FINAL COUNTDOWN: 6 to go

Treatment was ok today but, guys, I am getting fed up of this routine! Every day follows this basic routine: Wake up, meds, feel shattered, hospital, feel shattered, meds, bed.

Today I saw the yellow air ambulance helicopter land at the hospital. Exciting. I went swimming before hospital and after I finished hoovering my grandparents' house.

Question, after treatment as the radiographers take my mask off: (Me) 'I'm not going to do this [I felt it necessary to say this, why?] but if a patient turns up drunk do you have a right to refuse to treat them?' (Radiographers) 'Yes, mainly because they might fall off the bed!'

Lately this snack has brought me rapturous pleasure ... chicken and chips.

Wednesday September 10 2014

Treatment 25/30. FINAL COUNTDOWN: 5 to go

The treatment went fine and as it's number 25 I got some x-rays taken too. Treatment music today was excellent fun, 'The Dueling Banjos' – an absolute classic straight from hillbilly heaven.

Everything at hospital was late today. I forgot to take a snack with me and I got really hungry, bad plan. I don't always feel hungry any more like at the start of radiotherapy but if I start fixating on food I probably am. I realised I was when I caught myself staring at a lady eating a cereal bar. Laser beam eyes!

When I get that hungry, I get upset very easily. I had to go to my weekly review meeting; they asked me how I was doing and of course I got upset and said I was sick of radiotherapy. They said I'm doing really well and it's not long now. Well 'nuf said, not the most fun experience.

Thursday September 11 2014

Treatment 26/30. FINAL COUNTDOWN: 4 to go

Treatment went fine. No music. Gave the radiographers massive Yorkie chocolate buttons. I said to the Blonde Radiographer who is 21, 'You were born in the nineties' (WOW face). She said, 'So was she' (to a Brunette Radiographer, also 21). The Brunette Radiographer said, 'Oh no, do you think I look old?' I said, '23/24.'

After treatment I said, 'Don't feel bad because I think you're older than you are, it's because you both act so confident and professional.' The Brunette Radiographer said, 'That's a really good thing then.' I said, 'Enjoy your chocolate, thanks, bye.'

Question: (Me) 'If I'm not radioactive at any point after treatment why is my radiotherapy dose at its most potent a week after my treatment ends?' (Brunette Radiographer) 'Because its effects are cumulative, it's been building up all these weeks already and it is at its most effective a week after treatment. That's when we expect the most cell damage to be.' (Me speaking) 'I can accept that.' (Me thinking sarcastically) Awesome, can't wait.

I am a zombie, in the early part of radiotherapy the steroids I must take made me ravenous and I'd get painfully hungry really fast. But now those sneaky steroids have changed their ways; they still require me to eat loads of food but I don't always get hungry. I may need food and not feel it. Or I may become ravenous in a split second. Why does that make me a zombie? Because I wake up every time I want food, like a baby. I only sleep for an hour or 2 at a time.

Friday September 12 2014

Treatment 27/30. FINAL COUNTDOWN: 3 to go

Everything went fine. If you got the impression this whole thing is a bit less cruisey for me and more of a chore than in the first few weeks – you'd be right. But the end is so so so close.

    My bro Tom and his girlfriend Vanessa came to hospital today. After my mask had been fitted etc. they went to the radiotherapy office. Foot in mouth moment: my bro saw them working hard on computers and said he was surprised that they didn't just have to press GO. He was told that he could never return there. A joke with a hint of truth perhaps? I made pretty much the same blundering comment to the radiographers about a week ago when they explained to me what goes on in their office BUT I mitigated myself by *a.* being the patient they (perhaps) feel sorry for, *b.* Saying, 'I not saying you're stupid or anything but … I thought you might just come in here and press GO. I thought the treatment might have been programmed into your computer system by Dr A. Obviously your jobs are far more complicated than that.'

Monday 15th September 2014

Treatment 28/30. FINAL COUNTDOWN: 2 to go

I can't believe it, the end is so close! Today's musical offerings: Spice Girls, Tina Turner, All Saints. Easy listening, no complaints.

    One of the senior radiographers explained to me the hierarchy of assistant radiographers, junior radiographers, senior radiographers, superintendent radiographers, higher than that radiographers. It's a complicated system.

    Abi radiographer gave me a great idea of something to do with my mask after treatment has ended; the art college can't have it any more. I will make it into an ornament filled with fairy lights!

    Question: (Me) 'Have you ever started the radiation zapping and realised you've gone wrong?' (Radiographer) 'No, that's virtually impossible because we have so many checks to do before that.'

Still wearing shorts to treatment, it's supposed to be fairly nice weather this week so I think I'm gonna make it. I'm gonna wear shorts to all of my radiotherapy sessions.

Tuesday September 16 2014

Treatment 29/30. FINAL COUNTDOWN: 1 to go

Treatment went fine but I swear that face mask has got tighter; I'd blame this on my face getting a bit puffy because of the steroids I take. Treatment music was 'I Believe in Miracles' by Hot Chocolate; nice. Can I have a miracle please?

I spent nearly 3 hours in hospital today; it's draining. After radiotherapy I went to see my Symptom Support Dr (Dr H). We talked about recovery from radiotherapy; it's exciting, I can see big changes are coming. I am bored of going to hospital every day bla bla bla. The recovery period can take 6–8 weeks so Dr H said I can't go back to work just yet. However she encouraged me to swim regularly during my recovery to boost my general wellbeing and also to combat the bit of weight the steroids have made me acquire; they commonly do this to people.

I mentioned that gunk constantly comes out of my right ear to Dr H. She had a look then prescribed me some antibiotic ear drops to sort it out. So I have got one more med to take but it is not a tablet taken orally, it's ear drops. As of tomorrow I am looking forward to a reduction in the pills I have to take and Dr A (brain guy) will hopefully reduce my intake of steroids. Fingers crossed on this one please because they drive me crazy in a bad way.

Wednesday September 17 2014

Treatment 30/30!!!! It's the end!!!!

Music: they saved the best until last, The Ghostbusters Theme Song!! PHENOMENAL.

I actually feel like a huge weight has literally been taken off my shoulders. I am proud to announce that I wore knee-length shorts to every single one of my treatments – personal triumph!

I must say thanks to all the NHS staff for being friendly and professional. Today I gave my radiotherapy team cakes and sweets. All the radiographers have been so very lovely. And thank you to my mum for transporting me back and forth to hospital, even when I was grumpy.

As I'd hoped yesterday, Dr A is tapering me off steroids and I'll be off the little blighters totally by Oct 9 2014.

My advice if you ever need radiotherapy – prepare. Example 1: I love swimming so weeks before the treatment started I found out if I was allowed to do it, what guidelines I needed to follow regarding hygiene and then I made it happen. I found a local-ish pool that offered what I needed. Example 2: Stock up. I knew I would need emollient cream (E45) to put on my bald head patches, so I bought it ahead of treatment and then when I needed it, it was there. Example 3: Think about whose birthday will happen whilst you're being treated and buy their birthday present/card in advance. Example 4: (optional?) Get a meditation CD. Breathing meditation really helped me when I was face-jammed into that mask.

So now my course of radiotherapy is over what next? Just be yourself, everyone else is taken!

Somehow, radiotherapy has given me a great opportunity to re-evaluate my life and I conclude that in the future I will do more of what I want and less of what I don't care about.

I will have a few weeks/months to recover now but I feel it is appropriate to end this chapter here. I don't need to tell you all about my recovery and anyway I am entitled to a bit of privacy. I don't think it's necessary to tell you all that stuff as the emphasis of this final chapter is not my physical condition but how my mindset has affected proceedings throughout my course of radiotherapy treatment. However, if anyone does want to know how things worked out for me physically, feel free to send me an email (email address at the end of this book).

Back to Life

It seems relevant to write that by ending here I'm not robbing you of any magical ending, this situation is and always will be ongoing for me. I do have a brain tumour that I will have for the rest of my life. The purpose of this radiotherapy has never been to eradicate the tumour 100%; it is hoped to have significantly shrunk the beast and improved my eyesight, hearing, the functioning of my left leg, the motor coordination in my right hand, my balance and my coordination. However I won't find out the extent to which that has happened until I recover and get a brain scan later this year. In a few years' time it's entirely possible that I may need another form of treatment for my brain tumour, possibly chemotherapy.

What I feel it is important to convey to you through this chapter is that because of radiotherapy, I know who I am again. That has been given back to me in a way I never thought possible. And now I can think about the things I do and don't want to do. You can't if you don't know who you are.

I don't want to end by pretentiously telling everyone how to be positive, that would be irritating and fake. Everyone's life experience is precious, unique and totally incomparable to anyone else's. However I would urge anyone facing adversity to see it as an advantage and an opportunity to learn, not just a massive downer. I remained positive throughout my course of radiotherapy. I found that my attitude affected everything I experienced from emotional responses through to my physical organisation, like the amount I was willing to tidy my room. A few weeks before the treatment started I would never have predicted how positively I would face this challenge because I was completely terrified. However that positivity is and always has been deep down within me. For me, radiotherapy just gave it a chance to come out and re-educate myself about my own nature. That's why I said in my diary of treatment 12/30 (referring to radiotherapy) 'this is the best experience of my life', and I'm glad I said it because I mean it.

*Comments and general enquiries
to Emily Parr – realmofheroes@gmail.com*